W9-CLD-708

SPORTS INJURIES

Recent Titles in the Biographies of Disease Series

Parkinson's Disease
Nutan Sharma

Depression
Blaise A. Aguirre, M.D.

Diabetes
Andrew Galmer

Stroke
Jonathan A. Edlow

Autism
Lisa D. Benaron

Rabies
P. Dileep Kumar

Influenza
Roni K. Devlin

ADHD
Paul Graves Hammerness

Food Allergies
Alice C. Richer

Anorexia
Stacy Beller Stryer

Obesity
Kathleen Y. Wolin, Sc.D. and Jennifer M. Petrelli

SPORTS INJURIES

Jennifer A. Baima

Biographies of Disease
Julie K. Silver, M.D., Series Editor

GREENWOOD PRESS
An Imprint of ABC-CLIO, LLC

A B C C L I O

Santa Barbara, California • Denver, Colorado • Oxford, England

Library of Congress Cataloging-in-Publication Data

Baima, Jennifer A.
    Sports injuries / Jennifer A. Baima.
        p. cm. — (Biographies of disease)
    Includes bibliographical references and index.
    ISBN 978-0-313-35977-4 (hard copy : alk. paper) — ISBN 978-0-313-35978-1
(ebook) 1. Sports injuries. I. Title.
RD97.B35 2009
617.1'027—dc22   2009028094

13 12 11 10 9 1 2 3 4 5

This book is also available on the World Wide Web as an eBook.
Visit www.abc-clio.com for details.

ABC-CLIO, LLC
130 Cremona Drive, P.O. Box 1911
Santa Barbara, California 93116-1911

This book is printed on acid-free paper (∞)

Manufactured in the United States of America

Contents

Series Foreword

Every disease has a story to tell: about how it started long ago and began to disable or even take the lives of its innocent victims, about the way it hurts us, and about how we are trying to stop it. In this Biographies of Disease series, the authors tell the stories of the diseases that we have come to know and dread.

The stories of these diseases have all of the components that make for great literature. There is incredible drama played out in real-life scenes from the past, present, and future. You'll read about how men and women of science stumbled trying to save the lives of those they aimed to protect. Turn the pages and you'll also learn about the amazing success of those who fought for health and won, often saving thousands of lives in the process.

If you don't want to be a health professional or research scientist now, when you finish this book you may think differently. The men and women in this book are heroes who often risked their own lives to save or improve ours. This is the biography of a disease, but it is also the story of real people who made incredible sacrifices to stop it in its tracks.

Julie K. Silver, M.D.
Assistant Professor, Harvard Medical School
Department of Physical Medicine and Rehabilitation

Preface

I cultivated a love of sports medicine as a student athletic trainer for the University of Notre Dame from 1994 to 1997. Later, as a medical student and resident, I assisted with the medical care of collegiate athletes at Tulane University and Johns Hopkins University. Currently, I am a physician who is involved in caring for Boston area high school and recreational athletes. Often, it is hard for athletes to understand their injuries. When pain occurs, reason goes out the window. An athlete is trained to push harder, faster, better. In this book, I explain common sports injuries for those who are looking to learn more about this exciting area of medicine. Whether you are an athlete, want to go into the health care field, or are just interested in this topic, sports injuries are a fascinating area of medicine.

Acknowledgments

This book would not be possible without the following people. I would like to thank my patients, from whom I continue to grow and develop as a sports medicine physician. I would like to recognize my mentor, Dr. Barbara deLateur, who has always believed in the residents at Johns Hopkins Hospital. I appreciate the continued support of my colleagues, Dr. Zacharia Isaac and Dr Elinor Mody at Brigham and Women's Hospital and my chair, Dr. Ross Zafonte, at Harvard University Physical Medicine and Rehabilitation. I would like to recognize my parents, who started me on this great journey. Finally, I would like to thank Dr. Julie Silver for giving me this wonderful opportunity.

All photographs in this book were taken by Diane O'Brien. MRI and radiographic images come from the kind permission of the patients who experienced these injuries.

I would like to thank the Morse family—Jeff, Maureen, Jack, Peter, and Katherine—for posing tirelessly for photographs. I would like to thank Daphne Schmitt Boswell, Charles (Boz) Boswell, and Andy MacInnis for their enthusiastic participation in the sports photographs.

Introduction

K nute Rockne was head coach of the University of Notre Dame football team from 1918 to 1930. He coached the Irish for five undefeated seasons and led them to six national championships. His record includes 105 wins, twelve losses, and five ties. While working as a student trainer, I developed a great respect for and love of the football program at the University of Notre Dame. As one of the university's most successful and best-loved coaches, Knute Rockne popularized the forward pass. I chose to use his quotes in this book to illustrate that although much has changed since Rockne was a coach; the basic tenets of care of the athlete are the same. Play hard, have a great time, and we will be there for you when the game is over.

1

The History and Epidemiology of Sports Injuries

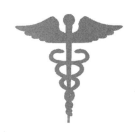

"Every team should have several comedians among them so that the squad is always in good humor. If my football squad is not laughing, sing-ing, or horse-playing in a shower bath I am alarmed. On the day of the game they should be raring to go and all on edge for the opening whistle."
—*Knute Rockne* (Rockne 1931, 12)

This quote captures the intense excitement at the beginning of the sporting contest. At the University of Notre Dame, the stadium would be filled to capacity and streaks of blue and gold paraphernalia would dot the stands. As student athletic trainers, we would have been up for hours filling the coolers and taping ankles. Amateur athletes of all ages would be tossing around the football all over the campus. During the first game of the season, the students would all be wearing the same shirt as if participating in a large-scale fashion faux pas. At the opening whistle, the resounding call would ring in my heart as it still does today ... "GO IRISH!"

Thoughts about sports in America evoke notions of football, basketball, golf, tennis, baseball, and soccer. These sports define seasons of the year and can bridge large television networks with a single tournament event. Although less publicized, sports also encompass activities from archery to orienteering, as well as a number of popular martial arts or a kayak race. As our information exchange has become more global, our access to knowledge of different sports has improved exponentially. For the purposes of this book, I will define sports as an event or activity, which involves individual or team participation in a competition of athletic talents.

The most widely recognized sports injuries occur in an instant when an athlete absorbs an unexpected blow. You've probably seen them on TV or online where the replay can be quite gruesome. Most people do not realize that sports injuries can also occur from repetitive use during the daily practice of any sport. Although it is the acute injury, especially when it's really devastating, that gets the most attention, awareness of common injury patterns will likely prolong an athlete's ability to enjoy sports participation. For example, the most common sports injury is ankle sprain. The chronic manifestation of this is lateral ankle instability, which involves weakness of the ligaments on the outside of the ankle. Often, this predisposes an individual to further injury. With proper care and treatment, sports performance need not suffer.

Although physical activity has always been part of the life cycle, the types of activities we perform have evolved with our society. When our society was purely agrarian, we used our physical strength to care for crops. Exercise outside of work was superfluous. As our society became more industrialized, our recreational pursuits evolved as well. In the nineteenth century, sports were viewed as purely recreation for the rich and famous. In the twentieth century, sports determined who was rich and famous, providing employment and entertainment. Now, we view sports both as a recreational outlet as well as an important part of a healthy lifestyle. Because most jobs currently involve less exercise, we have turned to sports to provide engaging ways to improve our health and fitness.

A rise in sports participation parallels our changing view of exercise. No longer a religious or a political movement, exercise promotion is championed by nearly every health care subspecialty. From cardiologists to psychiatrists, doctors are trying to get their patients to incorporate movement into their daily routines. Physical activity has become a necessary way to fight disease and prevent illness. Sports make physical activity fun and exciting. The thrill of competition encourages consistent practice and participation.

Even video games, such as the Wii from Nintendo, have evolved to simulate sports participation. These games used to simply involve clicking a mouse or moving a joystick. Now, they include foot pads that you can jump on or baseball bats connected to a computer cord.

THE OLYMPICS

The best-known sports competition, the Olympics, evokes a spirit of worldwide competition. Ancient Greeks began celebrating this five-day long festival in 776 BC. Initially, a stadium race was the only event of the games. Later, the festival included boxing, wrestling, and chariot racing. Even though the prize was a simple olive crown, winning athletes would be showered with gifts from their home city. Around the same time period, the Romans began chariot racing tournaments of their own. These two great societies not only shaped the development of tournament sports, they fashioned medical care as well. Galen, an ancient Greek physician and one of the fathers of medicine, began his career as a doctor to the gladiators.

The evolution of society prompted changes in both sports and medicine. There is little known about the care of athletes before the nineteenth century. Actually, most major advances came from the care of soldiers during times of war rather than the care of recreational athletes. Medical historians credit German society with the advances in medicine in the late nineteenth century that led to the birth of sports medicine. In fact, an estimated 40 percent to 50 percent of American medical students traveled to Germany or Austria to study in the last half of the nineteenth century. This is a staggering statistic given the expense and difficulty of travel in this time period. At this time, the first machine to measure the work of exercise was developed in Germany. This was called the ergometer. At the close of the nineteenth century, the creation of the first motor-driven treadmill followed. A greater understanding of exercise physiology followed from the ability to quantitate exercise. This is the foundation for how we train our athletes today.

A brief history of popular sports in the United States explains the evolution of sports medicine. Football remains the most popular sport in the United States. However, soccer holds the most popularity throughout the world. Remarkably, these two very different sports share a common history with most other ball game sports. Rounder and cricket, both early ball game sports, are likely the ancestors of our favorite sports. Although these are the best known ancestral ball game sports, few people know that there was a ball game sport in ancient Greece.

FOOTBALL

Harpaston was played on a field with goal lines similar to our modern-day football and included running down the field with the ball. Other countries lauded for the development of early football include China and Egypt. Eventually, this game evolved into the ball game played in England that we call rugby. Unlike in Ancient Greece, running with the ball was prohibited until 1823. In this year, a young player impulsively ran with the ball in his hands as the game was ending to make sure to score before time was up. This happy accident led to a change in the rules for the game and a commemorative stone for William Webb Ellis at the Rugby school in England.

Like the colonists, rugby traveled overseas to the New World. In the mid-1800s, several colleges and high schools played a rudimentary form of football. The first intercollegiate game occurred on November 6, 1869 between Rutgers and Princeton. This game was more like soccer than the football that we know today. A pivotal change occurred when Harvard played McGill University of Canada in 1874. The rules of both teams had to change to accommodate the other, and Harvard adopted a sport that was more like rugby. This was different than the games played at Princeton, Rutgers, and Yale, which were more similar to soccer. Eventually, Harvard convinced other intercollegiate teams, and the game evolved closer to what we now know as football. Like many great rivalries, Yale also claims they had the first "real" football team. Yale's first reported game may have been more like soccer, but they did have a famous doctor at the game. Ironically, he was not standing on the sidelines.

In a remarkable collision of sports and medicine, one of the founding fathers of American surgery played in the very first international football game in the United States. Yale University played against Eton College on December 6, 1873. (Eton was not an actual college, but a name for a group of Englishmen who wanted to play against the Yale team. Some of them had gone to a secondary school of the same name overseas.) The captain of the Yale team was William Stewart Halsted. Halsted was later recruited to be the first professor of surgery for the newly formed Johns Hopkins medical school. His legacy includes developing the first surgical residency training program in the United States, advancements in the accuracy of anatomic dissection, and innovative surgeries that incorporated applied physiology.

Football injuries can be devastating given that the game largely depends on the ability of very big men and boys to hurl themselves into each other. The rules and the equipment have changed greatly over the years to reduce injuries. Football involves colliding, catching, jumping, pivoting, running, and even kicking. Abrupt starts and stops predispose players to muscle strains. Collisions can result in injury to the nervous system. A common example of this is the stinger or burner. This is a brief shock to a collection of nerves that induces pain. Nerve pain has a radiating quality that feels like when the skin gets burned. These injuries usually resolve spontaneously and require little treatment other than sideline monitoring. If there is loss of sensation or muscle weakness, the player should be taken out of the game. The most catastrophic football injury is a brain or spinal cord injury. Although infrequent, these types of injuries can lead to confusion or even paralysis. Advances in collegiate and professional football rules and equipment have done much to prevent these serious sequelae.

SOCCER

Soccer's World Cup tournament is so popular that regional eliminations are held for more than a year just to determine what teams will earn the privilege of competition. In the third century, historical records indicate that soccer was played in England. The best theory is that this was introduced by Roman soldiers. Regardless, archery was the favorite sport of those in power due to its military application. Because soccer could not be rationalized as any form of military exercise, a ban was placed on the sport in the fourteenth and fifteenth centuries. Soccer was likely introduced to the United States in the nineteenth century.

Soccer could never be dubbed "as American as apple pie." Foreign nationals were the primary spectators and players of the game for seventy or eighty years. President Theodore Roosevelt tried to change this at the turn of the twentieth century out of concern for serious injuries and deaths that occurred as a result of American football. He spoke out against the dangerous nature of tackling, and encouraged Americans to take up soccer. This succeeded in changing the rules of the game of football rather than increasing participation in soccer. Soccer's popularity in the United States finally began to shift when the New York Cosmos recruited Pele out of retirement in 1975. With such a popular international figure on display, participation in both youth and adult soccer leagues increased dramatically. Today, soccer remains a favorite among children and their parents as the less dangerous cousin of football.

Since soccer involves little hand or shoulder use compared to football and baseball, common injuries tend to involve the lower limbs. Soccer players may have to pivot quickly and change direction. This type of movement can predispose a player to a ligamentous tear of the knee. Ankle injuries may occur with a wet soccer field, as this sport is usually played outside on grass. As more women are playing soccer, we have learned that these injuries can occur without player-to-player contact. Women and girls are more likely to sustain these noncontact ligamentous injuries while playing soccer for reasons we are still trying to understand.

TENNIS

Although now a country club favorite, tennis had crude beginnings as a sport where one attempts to swat the ball with his hand in an enclosed court.

Then, a glove was used to swat the ball. Eventually, a racquet followed. France exhibits records of the game of tennis as early as the thirteenth century. Tennis even shares responsibility for a history of gambling among the French and English nobility.

Although most sports arrived in the United States by way of England, Bermuda boasts more than the export of shorts to the United States. In America, tennis owes its origins to Mary Outerbridge. She saw the game in Bermuda in the late nineteenth century and arranged for a court to be constructed in New York. Eventually, the United States gained credibility in the game of tennis and became the location of a major tournament that hosts players from around the world. Despite the popularity of both men's and women's tennis, players were not compensated equally. Sports historians credit Billie Jean King, a famous female tennis player in the 1970s, with helping female athletes achieve cash prizes on par with those of male players.

There is an injury so common among tennis players that it is named for the sport. Tennis elbow, depicted in Figure 1.1, refers to chronic overuse that leads to tiny tears in the tendons on the outside of the elbow. This occurs because these tendons absorb great force when one is using a tennis racquet. These tendons are part of muscles that help extend the wrist. They span from the outside of the elbow to the back of the hand. In this age of computers, a

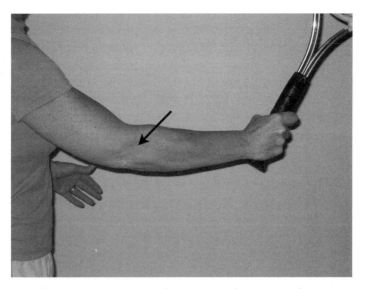

Figure 1.1. The tennis swing can result in too much stress on the wrist extensors. These muscles attach to the part of the elbow labeled in the figure, the lateral elbow. (Photo courtesy of Diane O'Brien)

similar overuse type of tendinopathy can occur with the repetitive wrist movements that are necessary for typing on the computer all day. Stretching can prevent both types of tennis elbow. The correct medical term for this is lateral epicondylitis. The lateral epicondyle is the outside part of the upper-arm bone called the humerus.

GOLF

Although it does not date back to the ancient Greeks, golf can claim a rich history. Alternatively promoted and banned by Scottish royalty, golf dates back to the fifteenth century. Scotland's ambivalent relationship with golf dissolved into a timeless love affair after the establishment of St Andrew's course in 1552. This course remains a popular vacation and tournament destination today with golfers from all over the world.

As with other European sports, players exported golf to the United States in the late 1800s. The victory of an American underdog popularized this sport. In 1913, Francis Ouimet, the son of a gardener and a Yankee, beat visiting European golf professionals in a famous tournament at The Country Club in Brookline, Massachusetts. Although the golf clubs may have changed from wooden to steel, you can still take in a round at The Country Club. A testament to the popularity of the sport, amateurs and professionals still study textbooks and videos today to get that perfect swing.

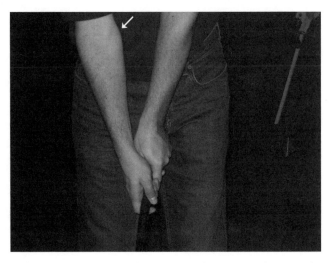

Figure 1.2. The golf swing can result in too much stress on the wrist flexors. These muscles attach to the part of the elbow labeled in the figure, the medial elbow. (Photo courtesy of Diane O'Brien)

The most common injuries that occur in golf may be those sustained by the ego. Golf is a fairly safe and controlled sport. There are no rapid actions, and the risk of contact injury is fairly low. The game can wait for each golfer to carefully line up for his swing. Since so much of the sport is about how you swing that club, the majority of the injuries come from this action. Like tennis, golf has an injury named for the repetitive motion that occurs in the golf swing. One can think of golfer's elbow as the opposite of tennis elbow. This occurs from the repetitive wrist flexion and pronation that is necessary in golf. Wrist pronation signifies turning the wrist palm down, as in putting your hand over an object. It is a chronic overuse injury of the tendons on the inside of the elbow. The medial epicondyle, labeled in Figure 1.2, is the location of pain in golfer's elbow.

BASEBALL

Even though the Super Bowl's enormous attendance has earned football the nickname of "the most watched" sport, baseball boasts the title of America's favorite sport. Although baseball shares some rules with its cousin cricket, Americans put their own spin on this popular sport. Granted, this included selling beer and paying the players. The English games of cricket and rounder are each thought to be the potential ancestor of baseball, and both were played in the Americas in the eighteenth century. In the nineteenth century, baseball clubs formed to allow for competition and establish rules. After we stopped battling each other in the Civil War, Americans got back to baseball. Ninety-one clubs attended the National Association of Baseball Players convention. This Association eventually dissolved, due in part to issues with gambling. By changing their tactics, those who made money from baseball founded other associations. The World Series was born when the two presiding leagues of baseball decided to play each other. Just the name of the tournament between these two American associations suggests that the United States had cornered the world market on baseball.

Baseball truly became a marketplace in 1920, when players from the Chicago White Sox were accused of taking money to lose the World Series in the previous year. The players were acquitted of charges, but excluded from playing again. This action helped to clean up the commonplace gambling in baseball, even among the players. Remarkably, in this period, a baseball player belonged to his team. The sale of Babe Ruth to the New York Yankees from the Boston Red Sox was one such historic example of this. Players did not earn their freedom to choose to switch teams of their own accord until the 1970s. Considering the staggering salary of the baseball players of the twenty-first century, it is hard to believe that only thirty years ago, the club owners had the advantage in wage determination. Today, the World Series has retained its name and popularity, but still involves only the two leagues in the United States.

Shoulder and elbow injuries have plagued Little League pitchers to the point where restrictions have been placed on players to prevent problems. Baseball requires a pitcher who can whiz the ball by the plate so fast that the opposing hitter has no opportunity to hit it. This action puts great stress on the muscles of the shoulder and elbow. Since children's bones are more fluid, this can result in a tiny chip of bone being pulled off the long bone by the connective tissue that attaches it to muscle. In adults, this same rapid and powerful shoulder motion can result in a tear of the muscles of the rotator cuff. This is why we commonly see the pitcher in the dugout with ice wrapped around his shoulder. We simply are not made to throw a ball faster than we can drive a car.

BASKETBALL

The most popular game in the United States may be football, and the favorite sport of Americans may be baseball, but only basketball can claim the United States as its birthplace. There is no doubt as to where basketball was born. However, some doubt that its creator acted alone. Dr. James Naismith developed the game to keep students entertained inside during the winter at Springfield Men's Christian Association Training School. Now called Springfield College, the school is still known for its physical education programs. The Basketball Hall of Fame still rests in basketball's birthplace of Springfield, Massachusetts. Basketball began at the professional ranks in the end of the nineteenth century. Since it is played indoors, it remains a popular sport long after our football and baseball seasons have ended.

Basketball is the most common sports activity during which players sustain injury. Basketball involves jumping up in the air while focusing on a basket that is above eye level, feet or yards away. It is extremely difficult to hit the basket while coming down solidly on two flat feet. Often, basketball players come down on one foot, on the side of one foot, or even on each other. Landing with a twisted foot causes stretching of the ligaments of the outside of the foot, also termed an ankle sprain. Fortunately, wearing an ankle brace can prevent this type of injury. The increased height of the sides of the sneakers used to play basketball was thought to help prevent the ankle from turning inward. In fact, wearing "hi-tops" does not prevent ankle sprain.

THE NUMBERS

The Centers for Disease Control and Prevention (CDC) estimates that high school athletes sustained 1.4 million injuries in the 2005 to 2006 school year (MMWR 2006). Researchers looked at nine popular high school sports to determine rates of injury in this year. Football players and wrestlers sustained the most injuries. The vast majority of these injuries were sprains and strains. When looking at the impact of these injuries, the sports during which athletes suffered the most devastating injuries were football, girls' basketball, and wrestling. Although girls' basketball had injury rates higher than boys' basketball, this difference was not large enough to be considered a significant finding.

Instead of choosing sports and looking at injury rates, researchers in another study (CONN 2003) asked patients what sports they played and how they got hurt. They interviewed patients of all ages, and found that those from ages five to twenty-four had the highest number of injuries. Basketball, football, and cycling resulted in the highest number of injuries in male patients. Exercising, gymnastics/ cheerleading, and basketball resulted in the highest numbers of injuries in female patients. Overall, the most frequently cited sport leading to injury was basketball. The most common sports injury in this study was sprain or strain. Ankle sprain is typically cited as the most common sports injury overall, although some experts report that the frequency of knee sprains may not take second place to that of ankle sprains.

2

Sports over the Life Cycle

"Injuries should receive instant attention. Of course we try to prevent them as much as possible. In the early scrimmages the players must be well protected as it is practice we want, we are not trying to beat anybody."
—*Knute Rockne* (Rockne 1931, 11)

Sports injuries vary widely depending on the age at which they are sustained. Developing bones have different needs than the fully formed skeletal system. Just as nutritional requirements are often different for children, injuries sustained are also different. In some ways, children are more resilient than adults and bounce back quickly from injury. In some ways, adults have the advantage because their skeletons are fully formed. This chapter will review the age-specific concerns in sports medicine.

CHILDREN (AGES 4 TO 14)

Children begin with sports that require low levels of hand–eye coordination and speed. "Child's play" is a common expression that denotes nothing serious or important. When children participate in organized sports, it can indeed become very serious. Children suffer different sports injuries than adults because their bodies are different. For the purposes of this book, children will be defined as those ages five to twelve. Of course, the sports activities of five-year-olds are far different from those of twelve-year-olds. Most children do not participate in organized competitive play until age five. By the age of twelve, children can be involved in organized practices before weekly games. Frequently, there may be a tournament at the end of the season that requires increased hours of play.

Young children often start out playing sports such as Tee ball and soccer. Tee ball is a modified form of baseball where the ball is set on a "T" or a modified traffic cone so that the inexperienced player can hit a motionless ball. Usually, this game is played by four- to six-year-old children. The goal is to progress to a moving target, as in baseball. Tee ball players number 2 million in the United States. That participation number jumps to 3 million when the players graduate to Little League. The United States Youth Soccer Association boasted 3.2 million registered players as of 2007. Although there is an effort toward organized sports in this age group, children often spend their leisure time riding bicycles. Actually, pedal cycling remains the most frequent cause of injury in children ages five to fourteen.

At the upper end of this age range, adolescence begins and changes in athletic performance are apparent. The length of the bones approaches that of the adult length. There are often marked differences in height and stature throughout middle schools in America. Teenagers develop at different rates. Ossification largely depends on pubertal development. Since there is great variation in onset and rate of puberty, this same variation applies to the growth and maturation of bone. Genetics determines part of this, but environmental factors such as intake of sugar steroids (called glucocorticoids) and amount and type of physical activity play an important role.

Children have bones that are still developing. Their bones are weak because they are not fully hardened or ossified. However, when a strong force is applied, something has to absorb the blow. Because bones are fully ossified in adults, the ligaments and tendons will often give first. In children, tendons are smaller and stronger. Thus, children are more prone to bony injury and adults are more prone to soft tissue injury when a force is applied in the same way.

We usually think of our skeleton as the strongest part of our body, since this is the framework for our bodies. In fact, some bones are not ossified until age twenty-one. The bones of the spine, called vertebrae, are a good example of late ossification. The growing bone is more susceptible to impact. The upside of this plasticity of bone is that children also usually heal faster. When a fracture is sustained in childhood, there is still a very good chance that there will be no long-term sequelae. When a fracture is sustained in adulthood, arthritis is likely to develop in that area. The ankle joint demonstrates the best example of this. Patients with hip and knee osteoarthritis may never have experienced trauma to these joints. In fact, obesity is often blamed as a major contributor to hip and knee osteoarthropathy, the degeneration of the protective tissue that covers the joint surfaces. When this occurs, contact of the worn surfaces produces joint pain. Since the joints of patients who are obese have to support a heavier load, this is thought to predispose these patients to osteoarthritis. In contrast, most patients who develop ankle osteoarthritis can identify a significant fracture or trauma that led to this phenomenon.

Differences in skeletal maturation and soft tissue compliance are a large part of the reason that children need different participation restrictions than adults. For example, many youth baseball pitchers experience shoulder and elbow problems affecting bones, ligaments, and tendons. Physicians evaluating these patients found that their injuries were usually related to overuse of the pitching arm. After much discussion, Little League established pitch counts to prevent such problems in these young athletes. Starting with the 2007 season, there is an upper limit placed on pitches per player per day. Currently, a thirteen- to sixteen-year-old player may pitch no more than ninety-five times per day. A player who is age seventeen or eighteen may pitch no more than 105 times per day. There are no such limits in place for major league baseball, but it is common practice to rotate pitchers in a single game, especially if one is performing poorly.

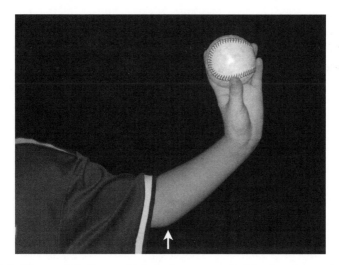

Figure 2.1. The medial elbow, which is the area marked in the picture above, is a common location of elbow pain in youth baseball pitchers. This pain often occurs in young players who start the pitch with their elbow too far forward. (Photo courtesy of Diane O'Brien)

ADOLESCENTS (AGES 14 TO 18)

In adolescence, the gap widens between boys and girls. Sports have long been considered a masculine endeavor. In contrast, femininity has not been associated with excellent athletic performance. The gender differences in athletic traits become more apparent in this age group as boys and girls develop their adult bodies. Boys excel in strength testing, especially in the upper extremities. In contrast, girls excel in flexibility. In this age group, gender bias develops in sports. Sports like football and gymnastics take advantage of the changes that occur during puberty. Football players are encouraged to visit the weight room to become big and strong. Female gymnasts are encouraged to push their flexibility as far as possible.

Current popular high school sports include football, wrestling, basketball, baseball, softball, volleyball, and soccer. Some high schools have hockey and field hockey. Although not usually offered in school, martial arts have become increasingly popular. Most Olympic gymnasts are still in high school when they compete. The pressure on these very young athletes is amazing. As the competition level increases, so do the injuries.

Adolescents face increasing demands for faster, better, and higher performance. These athletes have a more demanding training schedule than children. This increased activity is often not matched with an increased intake of nutrients. Adolescence is a time period recognized for its rebellion, which often involves poor nutrition. The junk food market is targeted toward adolescents. This perfect storm of increased athletic activity without a concomitant increase in nutrient intake may set the athlete up for bone metabolism problems in the future. This is particularly true in female athletes.

Women store the most calcium from ages eighteen to twenty-six. Calcium and vitamin D are the major building blocks for bone. Since osteoporosis (bone loss) is more common in women, female athletes who do not get proper nutrition as teenagers may be at a higher risk for bone loss later in life. The mechanism for this may be related to estrogen deficiency. Estrogen is stored in fat cells and regulates the menstrual cycle. When the composition of body fat goes too low, the patient stops having menstrual periods. The constellation of decreased nutrient intake, increased exercise, and menstrual irregularities is called female athlete triad. There is no corollary in male athletes.

As college costs skyrocket, many high school students view their sport as a ticket to a free education. The knowledge that college scouts may be in the audience or reading their hometown paper raises the level of competition. In sports such as football and baseball, this may have some dangerous consequences. Teenagers have utilized performance-enhancing drugs, such as anabolic steroids, to get ahead. Anabolic steroids are strength-building sex hormones, like testosterone. Although this was initially thought to be a problem confined to the boys' locker room, female athletes have tested positive for steroid use.

Initially, use of these drugs leads to rapid gains in strength. Complications of increased testosterone develop, such as mood swings, testicular atrophy, abnormal hair growth, high blood pressure, premature closure of the growth plates, and even liver tumors. What we know about steroids in high schools generally comes from surveys, as drug testing is not routinely performed. Mandatory drug testing begins at the collegiate level, except in the rare case of the high school athlete who happens to be an Olympian. The International Olympic Committee requires mandatory testing given the intense competition at this level of play.

YOUNG ADULTS (AGES 18 TO 22)

Young adults often enjoy such power contact sports as basketball, football, and soccer. Often, both scholarship and non-scholarship competition involves these sports. The National Collegiate Athletic Association (NCAA) sanctions many sports each season. In the fall, collegiate scholarship athletes may participate in cross country, field hockey, football, soccer, volleyball, and water polo. Of note, NCAA tournament-level volleyball is offered for female athletes in the fall and male athletes in the spring. Water polo is offered only for male athletes in the fall and female athletes in the spring. Winter sports offered include basketball, bowling, fencing, gymnastics, ice hockey, rifle shooting, skiing, swimming and diving, indoor track and field, and wrestling. The spring season brings baseball, golf, lacrosse, women's rowing, softball, tennis, outdoor track and field, and the return of volleyball and water polo for the opposite gender. Football and wrestling are the only sports offered for men only. Rowing and bowling are typically offered for women only. Of these sports, football and men's basketball generate the most revenue for colleges and universities.

The staggering amount of money generated from spectators of college football and basketball often goes to fund many other athletic and academic programs. In 2008, there were thirty-two bowl games. As a result of this revenue, $210 million was distributed to participating colleges and universities. Because the bowl championship series is not staged through the NCAA, it does not see the revenue. Reportedly, 90 percent of the NCAA's revenue comes from the men's collegiate basketball tournament, otherwise known as the Final Four. In the 2007 to 2008 season, the revenue was estimated at $614 million. Although this may be comparing apples to oranges, one can see that these two sports are major revenue sources. As a result, athletes and coaches of other sports complain that football and basketball receive all the attention and funding. Although this has led to some equipment envy among the teams, no one is complaining when the excess revenue trickles over to other programs or boosts enrollment of the school.

For those few lucky enough to achieve college scholarship play, their sport may keep them busy all year. For the rest of us, there are intramurals. The National Intramural-Recreational Sports Association offers campus championships in the following sports: soccer, flag football, soccer, tennis, and basketball. Although not one of your traditional sports, ultimate Frisbee is gaining popularity on college campuses. The Ultimate Players Association boasted 10,000 players in its 2008 collegiate championship series. Even if the sport does not have a championship, intramural college play is a great outlet for stress and a wonderful way to build leadership skills.

ADULTS (AGES 23 TO 65)

The shift from agrarian to industrial society greatly diminished required levels of physical activity. In adulthood, the focus of sports activity usually shifts to maintenance of weight or cardiovascular health. Few adults are required to perform heavy physical work every day. Machines have taken over most of the heavy lifting tasks. Most Americans have jobs that require desk work, such as sitting at a computer or answering phones.

This decrease in physical activity on a national level encouraged the government of the United States to develop the "Healthy People" series of objectives. Although these objectives also address disparities in health care, a major goal of this plan is to increase physical activity. For example, thirty minutes of moderate exercise for five or more days per week remains the recommendation for physical activity in this age group. In 1997, only 15 percent of adults met this recommendation. The government implemented a plan to raise this statistic to 30 percent of adults by 2010.

Unlike children, adults often enjoy solitary sports. Running is a popular adult sport because it involves little equipment or preparation. Going to the gym is another activity associated with adulthood. Most adults are aware that a balance between cardiopulmonary endurance exercise, such as running or biking, and strength training, as in weight lifting, offers the healthiest outcome. Like children, adults often enjoy the camaraderie of an exercise partner. From spinning class to running club, having a little encouragement from a partner or healthy competition from the group makes it that much easier to get frequent moderate exercise.

Adults may engage in sports with their young children that require intense cutting and running. This often leads to muscle strain or ligamentous sprain. Actions which may yield no pain in a child can plague the adult body. An older adult that goes up for a jump shot in basketball may be at risk for tearing the connection of the plantar flexors to the heel bone, called the Achilles tendon. An adult that pivots abruptly on a stationary foot while playing soccer may be at risk for an anterior cruciate ligament tear. These same actions are unlikely to cause injury in a child, whose soft tissues are more pliable.

SENIORS (AGES 65 AND OLDER)

Although cardiovascular health is important, the benefits of social interaction and mood elevation usually attract the senior athlete to continue sports participation. Seniors often enjoy sports such as tennis and golf. These sports require less repetitive ground contact and involve increasing amounts of technical skill. Despite the presumed slower pace of these sports, a significant benefit can still be achieved. Adults who participate in moderate exercise, regardless of the form, live longer lives than those who do not exercise. The cardiovascular benefits that come from exercise are thought to be responsible for this mortality benefit.

With the aging of the American population, osteoarthritis has claimed its place among important causes in the third millennium. Over 20 percent of the population of the United States reports some form of arthritis. Osteoarthritis is the breakdown of cartilage that leads to painful contact from worn joint surfaces. Activities that lead to repetitive joint loading can reproduce the pain. Initially, the pain might only occur with certain activities. Older athletes may need to avoid the harsh pounding that occurs with running or the potential collisions in contact sports. Eventually, the cartilage may degenerate leaving exposed bone. This contact of exposed weight-bearing surfaces can cause pain, even with walking.

We used to discourage activity in this age group as we thought it would worsen the pain of osteoarthritis. Actually, moderate exercise has a protective effect on osteoarthritis. Patients who exercise regularly achieve improved outcomes in regard to function and pain. This phenomenon is likely related to improved function of the immune system and mood with exercise as well as the protective effect of stronger muscles and more flexible soft tissues. Exercise may become even more important after joint replacement surgery.

When patients suffer from advanced arthritis, joint replacement is recommended. This is graded by both radiographic evidence of joint degeneration as well as a decrease in the patient's physical activity level. Currently, most patients with hip and knee replacements do very well. Hip and knee osteoarthritis is very common, and these joints have a fairly reproducible arc of motion. Shoulder replacement techniques have become more promising with each passing year, but the motion left is still limited compared to what a native shoulder can perform. Currently, there are no widely accepted elbow or ankle replacement devices. As joint replacement products evolve to replicate normal motion, surgeons are decreasing activity limitations on patients after joint replacement. The number of athletes with replacement parts remains on the rise, and we are learning more every day about their capabilities.

GENDER

Women are more likely to get mild ankle sprains than men. Female athletes get more knee sprains than male athletes. Because women suffer more ligamentous injuries than men, presumably women have more laxity in their ligaments. Several theories exist to explain this phenomenon. One theory is that increased estrogen levels result in more laxity and increased injury. Of note, women do not have an increased incidence of ligamentous tear at the point in their menstrual cycle when their estrogen is highest. Also, exogenous estrogen intake occurs when women take oral contraceptives. However, women on oral contraception do not have more ligamentous tears.

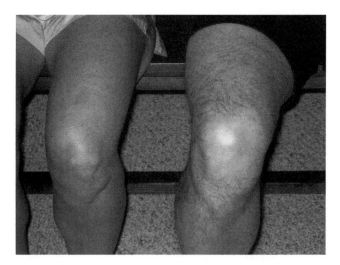

Figure 2.2. Compare the appearance of the anterior knee of a woman and a man. The male knee is on the right. Note the more prominent and toned appearance of the male quadriceps as compared to the female quadriceps. (Photo courtesy of Diane O'Brien)

Another theory involves the biomechanics of a woman's body. Women are built differently than men. Women have wider hips than men. Their knees are in a more valgus (inward pointing) position. Generally, they have weaker quadriceps and hamstring muscles. This relative muscle weakness may be related to a mechanical disadvantage given the slightly different biomechanics or to the hormonal changes that occur during puberty.

As previously mentioned, boys develop increased strength as compared to girls during puberty. Although this is far more apparent in the upper limbs, there is a discrepancy in lower limb strength as well. In particular, boys tend to have stronger hamstrings than girls. The quadriceps to hamstring ratio is known to be five to three in adult males. This ratio is thought to be skewed more toward the quadriceps in women, on the order of six to three. For this reason, programs for the prevention of anterior cruciate ligament tear in women focus on hamstring strengthening. Since these muscles are knee flexors, exercises that involve squats or lunges are recommended.

3

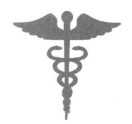

Common Sports Injuries

"Charley horses are of two kinds: first, the one produced by hard impact; second, a sprained or pulled muscle, caused by stopping suddenly. The one caused by hard impact is a bruised muscle and blood is allowed to escape into the surrounding tissue. The best cure for this is a massage and heat ... In the case of the second type of charley horse the athlete should have the area taped tightly then be let off for a week or two."
—*Knute Rockne* (Rockne 1931, 12)

Some older patients use the term charley horse to refer to a muscle pain. In the first case, Rockne is referring to a collection of blood in a muscle called a hematoma. Initially, we treat every sports injury with ice for at least the first twenty-four hours. The reason for this is that heat worsens bruising and swelling by increasing blood flow to the area. Ice causes the blood vessels to constrict. This decreases the surrounding swelling and bleeding. After the bleeding has stopped, heat can be used to help with stiffness. Massage can certainly be helpful for sore muscles.

We still tape our athletes for both treatment and prevention of injury as Rockne recommended for the treatment of the second type of charley horse. In the twenty-first century, we use more prefabricated braces to protect the injured part, but the concept of splinting remains the same. The injury should be immobilized in the position of function and the athlete should be put out on injured reserve until he or she demonstrates pain-free activity. For a muscle strain, seven to fourteen days remains a reasonable recommendation.

Though the field of sports medicine has grown since Rockne's days, many of these basic treatment recommendations have changed very little.

PAIN GENERATORS

There is a whole collection of nerves simply dedicated to carrying pain signals from the periphery. Consequently, nerves are often thought of as the main pain generators in the body. These are sensory nerves. In fact, there are many structures that could potentially cause pain after injury. Motor nerves feed the muscles. When they are not working, the muscles become weak. However, nerve injury is not the only reason for muscle weakness. Local muscle injury or pain alone can cause weakness. This convergence of possible reasons for muscle weakness makes the physical exam and imaging modalities nearly as important as the patient's history in determining the diagnosis.

Nerve pain is often characterized by complaints of burning, radiating, or numbness and tingling. Nerve pain can occur if the nerve is cut or stretched during a trauma, is pinched by surrounding structures, or becomes sick. Sickness of the nerves or "neuritis" may be from environmental toxins, nutritional deficiencies, or viral pathogens. We can check blood tests for some of the toxins and most of the nutritional deficiencies, but we do not have good tests for viruses. Diabetes is another common reason for nerve dysfunction in the United States. If a patient has diabetes, it is much harder to tell if there is a nerve injury in addition to the diabetes. Not only do nerves connect to muscles, they feed the bones as well.

With fracture, acute severe pain occurs due to the insult to bone. Swelling and bleeding may cause pain just by taking up space in a place where there was no room for extra fluid. Soft tissue, such as tendons, ligaments, meniscus, and joint capsules can also cause pain. Tendons attach muscle to bone. When a muscle belly is torn, often a bruise is present on physical exam. Ecchymosis does not often occur with partial tendon tear. Ligaments connect bone to bone. Loss of continuity of a ligament may result in pain and instability. Tearing of connective tissue can result in many different symptoms, depending on the severity and location of the injury.

Inflammation is another source of pain. Swelling, warmth, or erythema on physical exam or increased fluid on magnetic resonance imaging (MRI) suggests inflammation. The suffix—itis—is used to denote this phenomenon. For example, tendinitis is used to describe inflammation of the tendon and bursitis to denote inflammation of the bursa. A bursa is a fluid-filled sac that is present in normal individuals. It functions to help tendons glide more smoothly and becomes painful only when inflamed. Since a patient can have tendonitis and bursitis at the same time, it may difficult to determine the primary pain generator.

The patient's story of how the pain began weighs heavily in the diagnosis of sports injury. For example, a patient who turned his or her ankle while running nearly always has an ankle sprain. A soccer player who stubs his or her toe likely has turf toe. Traumatic injury is often more worrisome than pain without an inciting trauma. Fracture is higher on the list of possible diagnoses in this case. Certain common patient complaints are very suggestive of specific musculoskeletal injuries. Patients who complain that the shoulder hurts to sleep on nearly always have subacromial bursitis. Patients who cannot straighten the knee often have excess fluid in the joint. Patients with clicking or locking of the knee joint may have a meniscal tear.

An accurate description of aggravating and relieving factors helps us determine the possible pain generator. For example, tendinitis or bursitis pain is often worse with pressure over the area or with activities that require shock absorption, such as jumping or running. Muscle pain is typically worse when activating the injured muscle. Arthritis pain is a dull ache that is worse when bearing weight through the joint. It is often associated with stiffness. Nerve pain is not localized to the weight-bearing surfaces of a joint. It often radiates down the limb in the distribution of the injured nerve and may be accompanied by numbness.

The patient's description of pain limits the physical exam to the area of potential pathology. Key components of the musculoskeletal exam include inspection, palpation, range of motion, strength and sensory testing, and special provocative tests. On inspection, we are examining the skin for clues to the etiology of pain. If there is a break in the skin, infection becomes suspect as there is now a means of entry for bacteria. If there is a rash, this could be completely coincidental or related to the patient's current musculoskeletal problem.

Two rashes that typically cause pain are erythema migrans and herpes zoster. Erythema migrans is a red rash in the shape of a circle with a large central clearing that signifies Lyme disease. Lyme disease can cause arthritis in a joint or irritation of a nerve. The treatment of Lyme disease is antibiotics. Herpes zoster is the medical term for the shingles, which is a form of chicken pox. This rash looks like tiny bubbles on the skin with fluid inside. Since the virus lives in a spinal nerve, it follows the same pattern on the skin that the nerve would take to innervate the skin. This pattern is called a dermatome.

The pain may occur before the rash, but after two weeks of pain the rash will be present if the diagnosis truly is herpes zoster. The treatment of herpes zoster is antiviral medicine. Of note, antibiotics work better than antivirals because bacteria don't have the ability to change to survive. Since viruses can mix up their genetic codes, they can outlast the antiviral medication. For this reason, antibiotics tend to end an illness and antivirals simply shorten the duration of the illness.

Palpation may be the most important part of the musculoskeletal exam. Initially, the skin is touched lightly to judge the patient's sensitivity to touch in the area of their injury. Once trust is achieved, deeper palpation can be performed to determine the location of the worst pain. Knowledge of anatomy is essential to understanding the results of sensitivity to touch. If the tenderness is over a bony prominence, there may be a fracture or a bone spur. If the tenderness is over a muscle, there may be muscle spasm or tendinopathy. Some joints are easier to palpate than others. For example, the shoulder joint is rather superficial when palpating from the front or the side of the patient. The hip joint is buried under significant soft tissue and even careful palpation has little diagnostic yield. There are only three places that the nerves become superficial to palpate. In the front of the wrist, the median nerve can sometimes be felt as it passes through the carpal tunnel. The peroneal nerve may be felt as it winds around the outside of the knee. The ulnar nerve may be felt as is passes around the medial epicondyle. The medial epicondyle is called the funny bone because of the ulnar nerve. When one hits his elbow over this area, the pain can travel all the way down the inside of the arm into the ring and pinky fingers resulting in this "funny" sensation.

Another important component of the musculoskeletal exam may be a range of motion exam, which involves putting the joint through all of the normal motions it should have and comparing that to what the patient can actually do. Passive range of motion is what the examiner can demonstrate with the patient's joint. Active range of motion is what the patient can perform independently. For example, abduction of the shoulder is lifting the arm up with the palm of the hand facing forward. This action is largely supported by the muscles of the rotator cuff. If the patient can only get halfway through the motion and the examiner can get the arm all the way up, this is a sign of muscle weakness. If the patient can only get halfway way up and the examiner cannot get the shoulder up any higher, this is a sign of joint contracture or formation of fibrotic soft issue that prevents joint motion.

Muscle weakness signifies muscle tear or motor nerve injury. Strength testing challenges the muscles. A muscle cannot generate much force when it is stretched to capacity. It exhibits the most force when it is between fully stretched and fully lax. It is at this midpoint that we typically test the muscles. However, if the patient is a very strong male body builder and the examiner is a tiny female doctor, she can use this concept of muscle strength versus length to her advantage. For example, leg muscles are larger and stronger than arm muscles in normal patients. Since the examiner has to use her hands to examine the patient's legs, she can put the leg muscles at a greater angle to test for subtle changes in strength. Another way to apply this concept is through the use of gravity. Asking the patient to walk on the toes is more likely to bring out subtle weakness than having the patient step on the examiner's hand while seated. Although both actions test the ankle plantar flexors, gravity will always be able to exert more force on these muscles than the examiner can generate with her hand.

It is imperative to know whether sensory loss is present as this is highly suggestive of nerve injury. There are several components to sensation, such as sensitivity to touch, pain, temperature, and position sense. Different components are present in different pathways in the spinal cord, but the pin prick exam provides a good indication of the presence of sensory loss. This exam is performed by using a paperclip, safety pin, or monofilament to press against areas of potential concern. This is compared to the same area on the uninvolved limb. If the patient describes a decreased ability or an inability to feel the instrument, this is described as sensory loss. The pattern of sensory loss may determine the injured nerve. For example, if the ulnar nerve is injured at the elbow, then there will be decreased sensation in the ring and pinky fingers of the hand. Special tests for musculoskeletal injury will be discussed under the heading for the joint that they are used to assess.

SHOULDER

The shoulder joint can perform an impressive arc of motion. The shoulder joint looks like a large ball that does not fit its socket. Some doctors liken this joint to a golf ball on a tee to illustrate this concept. Just like a golf ball, the humerus is much larger than its tee, the glenoid fossa. The only thing that holds this golf ball on the tee is a band of fibrocartilage called the labrum and a group of muscles called the rotator cuff. The advantage to this conformation is the ability to rotate the shoulder in many planes, as occurs in pitching a baseball. The disadvantage is that the shoulder can dislocate much easier than the other joints.

The bones of the shoulder include the humerus, the clavicle, and the scapula. The humerus is the large long bone that forms the upper part of the arm. This bone contains the "ball" part of the socket. The clavicle, otherwise known as the collar bone, is the horizontal bone in the front of the shoulder.

The scapula is the bone often called the shoulder blade. The scapula forms the true shoulder joint, or glenohumeral joint, by articulating with the humerus at the glenoid fossa. The glenohumeral capsule covers this joint. A complex of ligaments arises from the front of the joint capsule and serves to stabilize the shoulder joint. The scapula forms the acromioclavicular (AC) joint by articulating with the clavicle at the front of the shoulder. Three ligaments, named for the segments of the bone that they connect, lend stability to this joint.

Dislocation of the true shoulder joint is not a subtle injury. The ball of the humerus slides out in front of the glenoid fossa. When this happens, the ball part of the joint forms a large bulge in the wrong place. The ball usually pops out forward, but in more rare instances can pop out toward the back. A compression fracture, called a Hill-Sachs lesion, may occur when the head of the humerus makes contact with the front of the glenoid. This results in a fracture of the back part of the humeral head and usually occurs when the humerus dislocates in a forward (anterior) motion. Evaluation after dislocation always includes radiographs to look for associated injury to bone. The shoulder joint is the most vulnerable when one is reaching out and up, as if in pitching a ball. If an athlete has loose ligaments or sustains a blow in this position, the humerus can dislocate and cause subsequent soft tissue damage. Although the labrum does not contribute to the muscle power of a throw, it does help to stabilize the joint by forming a circle around the glenoid. When dislocation results in a tear of the front of the labrum, this is called a Bankart lesion.

Dislocations of the true shoulder joint can result in injury to the ligaments or tendons. The glenohumeral ligaments, together with the joint capsule and the labrum, stabilize the shoulder joint. Sprains occur when these ligaments are disrupted, but not torn. Shoulder dislocation injuries may involve strains, as tendons attach to the large rounded portion of the humerus. Both always involve deformity, either due to loss of connective bands of tissue or the force of a muscle that had previously been counterbalanced. For example, when the supraspinatus is torn, the humerus is often pulled upward due to the superior force of the deltoid that is now no longer balanced by the rotator cuff. Edema is usually apparent and may obscure the clinical exam. MRI may be helpful to visualize exactly what soft tissue has been injured with the dislocation.

Although not a common injury, shoulder dislocation can be painful and debilitating when it occurs. It always needs to be treated with reduction. Reduction involves putting the joint back into place. Usually, this can be done without surgery with gentle traction on the shoulder or the use of weights. It is best performed by a trained professional as it can be excruciating for the patient. If done incorrectly, it can cause further injury to the bones, muscles, or nerves. If the shoulder is not reducible, then surgery is necessary.

The most common shoulder sprain occurs when the clavicle gets separated from the acromion, or the upper part of the shoulder blade. An AC separation results from a tear of the acromioclavicular (A) or coracoclavicular (C) ligament or both. Instead of popping out to the front like the humerus, the two sides of the joint get pulled apart from each other in a horizontal plane. The acromioclavicular and coracoclavicular ligaments may be torn with acromioclavicular joint sprain. The acromioclavicular ligament is the first to be injured. This may occur even with the mildest sprain. Injury to the coracoclavicular ligament indicates a larger problem and results in deformity of the collarbone. When a sprain is serious enough to tear the coracoclavicular ligament, the collarbone pokes backward into the trapezius muscle, resulting in a visible depression in the front of the shoulder.

This injury happens after a direct impact to the shoulder, as in shoulder-to-shoulder contact during a football game. Falling on an extended arm can also lead to AC separation. On physical exam, there is a small depression in the front of the shoulder at the area of separation. This separation of the joint can be visualized on radiographs. Associated small fractures can be seen using computed tomography (CT). Often, an MRI is not needed as diagnosis of related soft tissue injury does not usually change treatment.

Treatment depends on the degree of the sprain (graded I to VI depending on severity) and the patient's occupation or sport. Most AC injuries can be treated with rest, ice, activity modification, and physical therapy. For severe sprains, surgery can repair the joint by fixing the two bones together or with resurfacing of the distal clavicle and reconstruction of the coracoclavicular ligament. The activity level of the patient is also important when deciding on treatment options. For example, a forty-year-old man who does manual labor for his job may pursue surgical repair, whereas an eighty-year-old woman would be unlikely to elect this option as the potential risks of surgery might outweigh the benefits.

Strain of the rotator cuff or rotator cuff tendinopathy is the most common sports injury of the shoulder. The rotator cuff is made up of the supraspinatus, infraspinatus, teres minor, and subscapularis muscles. These muscles all work together so that one can throw a ball. The supraspinatus helps to raise the shoulder when the arm is by the side. The infraspinatus and the teres minor help to reach backward over the head as in cocking the ball. The subscapularis helps to turn the shoulder in when pitching forward. For this reason, rotator cuff tendinopathy or tear is common in ballplayers. Some physicians refer to the biceps muscle as the fifth rotator cuff muscle. This muscle courses from the humerus and the scapula (at the coracoid) to the elbow. Pain from tendinopathy of this muscle is difficult to separate from pain of the rotator cuff muscles, as it occurs at the very same location in the body.

The supraspinatus is the most commonly torn rotator cuff muscle. Since this muscle helps reach up over the head (termed abduction), this motion is very painful with a torn supraspinatus. The infraspinatus, which internally rotates the shoulder, is often the next muscle to be torn. The subscapularis and teres minor may be involved, but to a lesser extent than the other muscles. Often, we will examine patients by having them bring their arms up to the side of their head and then slowly lower them down as in an arc. If a patient is unable to do this, it is a called a positive painful arc test and is a sign of rotator cuff tear. Although we can tell that a tear is likely present, this test does not tell us which muscle is torn.

Physical exam tests can sometimes isolate which muscle is causing the pain. The examiner will often try to isolate the different muscles by strength testing each one individually. When a patient is in a pain, the strength exam is often limited. The Neer and Hawkins tests are commonly used to assess for rotator cuff tendinopathy in any of the muscles. The Neer test involves bringing the patient's arm up by the side with the palm facing down, as depicted in Figure 3.1. The Hawkins test involves abducting and internally rotating the shoulder. This test should be performed in several planes to best assess for impingement.

Either test is positive if it elicits pain in the anterolateral shoulder. In the empty can test, the patient is asked to act as if holding cans of soda out in front of her and then turn the cans upside down. This test is supposed to

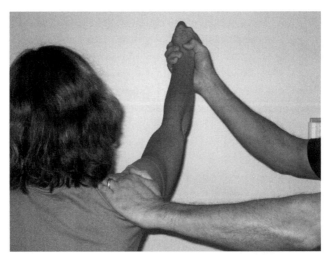

Figure 3.1. Neer's test involves stabilizing the shoulder blade with one hand and bringing the affected arm up towards the head with the other hand. Pain in the front or side of the shoulder indicates a positive test. (Photo courtesy of Diane O'Brien)

isolate tears of the supraspinatus muscle. To test the subscapularis muscle, the patient is asked to reach up the back toward the shoulder blade with the palm facing outward. In this position, the patient must lift the hand off the back. If the patient cannot perform this action, then the subscapularis is torn. Access to MRI has revolutionized our ability to assess the rotator cuff. MRI can not only establish the injured muscle or muscles, but it can assess the extent of the injury as well.

Tendons can be irritated, inflamed, or worn. Most doctors now use the term tendinopathy to refer to pain at the insertion site of muscle. We used to use the term tendinitis as we thought the pain was from inflammation around the tendon. However, advanced imaging techniques have shown us that inflammation is not always present with tendon pain. Currently, we think the pathology reflects microscopic tears in the tendon. (In more severe cases, tendons can be torn through as well. Tendon tear can result from a single sharp blow or fall on an outstretched hand.) Tendinopathy occurs when an athlete uses these muscles too much or in an unhealthy way. This is far more common than full-thickness tendon tear.

Unlike with biceps tendinopathy, a biceps tear can be distinguished from a supraspinatus or infraspinatus tear. These rotator muscles reside on the back of the shoulder and insert on the front. Although the biceps begins in essentially the same place that the rotator cuff ends, it inserts on the elbow. A torn biceps will often result in a visible or palpable bulge on the front of the upper arm. This has been termed a "Popeye" deformity because of the awkward and easily visible appearance of the torn muscle. A torn supraspinatus or infraspinatus creates a more subtle deformity at the back of the shoulder, which is much harder to detect on physical exam.

The four rotator cuff muscles and the biceps attach in the area of the subacromial bursa. The bursa can become inflamed independently, but bursitis is often seen in conjunction with tendinitis. Diagnosis is made either with local tenderness over the bursa or with increased fluid seen in the bursa on MRI. Since it is so interrelated with the tendinitis, it is treated in a similar fashion. The inflamed bursa responds best to interventions that decrease the inflammatory cells in the fluid, such as ice, anti-inflammatories, and local steroid injection. Once the pain is improved, physical therapy is prescribed to correct the underlying biomechanical deficit that may have led to the bursitis.

Sometimes, rotator cuff injuries are related to poor throwing mechanics and sometimes this is simply from performing overhead activities with a frequency that the shoulder cannot tolerate. The only way to sort this out is to observe the patient's shoulder mechanics and make corrections. A physical therapist can help an athlete train other muscles to assist the rotator cuff in throwing and improve overhead activities. An important component of healing the ten-dinopathy involves limiting the activity of these muscles that can be achieved with a break from the sport or with limitations on the frequency of the action. This concept of activity limitation led to the pitch counts developed for Little League mentioned in the previous chapter. Volleyball and swimming are other sports where overhead activity limitation becomes a concern in sports medicine.

If the rotator cuff is torn completely through or a partial tear does not respond to physical therapy, surgery may be recommended. Repair of the rotator cuff involves reattaching the torn tendons. If the bursa is swollen or the labrum is torn, these areas may be cleaned up. If there are bone spurs, called osteophytes, from arthritis, these may be shaved. Rotator cuff surgery can be done open or with arthroscopy. Open surgery is the older form of surgery which involves a large scar, but allows the surgeon to clearly visualize and access the shoulder joint. Arthroscopic surgery is when tiny incisions are made allowing a scope to pass through. The scope has a small camera on the end which sends an image to a television screen. Fluid is pumped into the joint to allow for improved visualization. Tools are inserted through the tiny incisions to make repairs. Most patients prefer this type of surgery since the incisions are smaller and the recovery time is less. The type of surgery elected depends on the extent of the injury.

If the shoulder pain that occurs from rotator cuff tendinopathy, tear, or bursitis is left untreated, frozen shoulder may develop. Frozen shoulder refers to scarring of the shoulder capsule and fibrosis of the soft tissues that affects the shoulder range of motion. The medical term for this is adhesive capsulitis. This condition is the result of a vicious cycle. The patient experiences shoulder pain. It hurts to lift the arm up, so the patient holds the arm close to the body. In a few weeks, the patient is no longer able to lift the arm up. This condition is difficult to treat and requires aggressive stretching. If the stretching does not work, surgery can be done to cut away the adhesions. The trouble with surgery for scar tissue is that it often comes back. For this reason, adhesive capsulitis is best prevented in the first place. Prevention involves early range of motion and analgesia after shoulder injury.

Adhesive capsulitis rarely occurs in young athletes because they are often more aggressive about rehabilitation and their soft tissues tend to heal more quickly. This condition usually occurs in middle-aged athletes. It happens more often in women than men for reasons we do not understand. It happens more often in diabetics because their tissues heal more slowly. Patients with underlying abnormalities of the ball part of the socket are also at a higher risk. Diagnosis involves not only the patient's inability to raise the arm above the shoulder, but also the examiner's inability to raise the patient's arm. Radiographs should be done to check for bone injury or deformity. Prompt physical therapy is the mainstay of treatment.

Often, the physical therapist will use ultrasound to help ease the pain and allow for tissue healing prior to initiating a stretching program. Initially, the stretching program will involve Codman's exercises. These exercises are performed with the patient bent over at the waist and the arm hanging down toward the floor. Gravity is used to initiate subtle pendulum-like rotations of the affected limb. As the patient improves, larger circles can be traced with the frozen shoulder. Eventually, these circles can be performed with the patient upright. Encouraging the patient to stand upright and walk his fingers up a wall to the highest level they can achieve is called wall-walking, which is another stretching exercise to treat or prevent frozen shoulder.

Another shoulder problem that generally occurs only in older athletes or those with rheumatologic disorders is arthritis. Arthritis is when the cartilage covering the bone breaks down and leads to pain. There are two main types of arthritis: osteoarthritis and inflammatory arthritis. Osteoarthritis is the degenerative or wear-and-tear arthritis that can come from previous trauma in an area or from age-related changes of the joint. Inflammatory arthritis is an autoimmune disease. The body recognizes its own joint cells as foreign and starts breaking down these cells through the immune system. This is similar to the process that occurs when the body fights bacteria. However, the joints are not infected with a foreign organism. A mistake in the recognition process of the immune system leads to dysfunction and subsequent attack of one's own joints. Either type of arthritis can lead to pain in the shoulder joint. When the patient has trouble with combing her hair or brushing her teeth due to this pain, shoulder replacement is usually recommended.

Shoulder replacement surgery takes about two to three hours and requires a hospital stay of two to three days. A prosthetic shoulder may last up to fifteen years. A partial shoulder replacement means that the surgeon has put in a metal ball to replace the rounded portion of the humerus, but left the socket part of the joint alone. A partial shoulder replacement is a good option for fractures of the humeral head or problems that have only affected this bone. When arthritis affects both the ball and socket of the glenohumeral joint, then a total shoulder replacement is the best option. A new cup is installed over the glenoid and a new ball replaces the humeral head. The range of motion after shoulder surgery depends on the type of shoulder problem and the healing of the overlying musculature.

Another potential source of shoulder pain is from a relay station of nerves under the collarbone. Fortunately, this plexus of nerves is well buried so as to avoid injury. The brachial plexus forms from individual nerves that exit the spinal cord at the cervical segments. Two individual segments join together to form the upper trunk and two join together to form the lower trunk. The nerve in the middle, labeled C7, becomes the middle trunk. These trunks then branch further providing a complex network. At the level of the collarbone, these nerves join together again in a different pattern.

Nerve injury can occur anywhere along the pathway. In general, it requires a significant trauma to damage the brachial plexus. Permanent brachial plexus injury can result from birth trauma or a fall from a height. Temporary injury may occur with shoulder-to-shoulder contact in sports. The burner or stinger described in football is from nerve pain due to trauma to the brachial plexus. This pain is usually self-limited and resolves spontaneously. If there is any residual sensory or motor deficit, the athlete should be removed from play until further studies can be done.

Sometimes, it is difficult to determine if the injury is at the level of the nerves as they exit the spine or at the shoulder where they dive down deep under the clavicle. One physical exam maneuver to determine this is to extend the patient's neck. This is called the Spurling maneuver, and it results in reduced room available for the nerves to course out of the spine. Testing of the right-sided nerve by Spurling maneuver is depicted in Figure 3.2. If there is any mechanical compression at the level of the spine, the patient will experience worsening of pain with this test. If it is at the shoulder, there will be no change in pain with neck movements. A more scientific way to check the nerves is with electromyography. This procedure is further described in Chapter 4.

After the brachial plexus forms into the medial, posterior, and lateral cords at the collarbone, it divides even further to individual nerves. Individual nerves that can cause shoulder problems when injured include the suprascapular nerve, the axillary nerve, the long thoracic nerve, the dorsal scapular nerve, and cranial nerve eleven. The suprascapular nerve branches off the upper trunk of the brachial plexus and feeds the supraspinatus and infraspinatus muscles of the rotator cuff. This nerve can become injured where it courses over the top of the shoulder blade during overhead sports or when a back pack is worn for long periods of time. Injury to this nerve at the top of the shoulder blade results in weakness of both of these important rotator cuff muscles. At the level of the middle of the shoulder blade, suprascapular nerve injury results in weakness of the infraspinatus only, which functions in shoulder external rotation.

The axillary nerve innervates the teres minor and the deltoid muscle, a large muscle responsible for raising the shoulder. Although not part of the rotator cuff, the deltoid provides a large proportion of the strength of the shoulder. The axillary nerve branches off of the posterior cord of the brachial

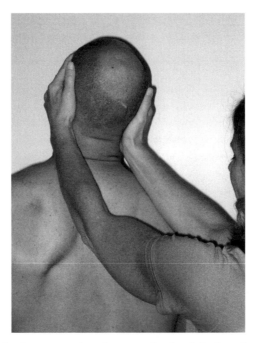

Figure 3.2. Spurling's test involves bringing the head backwards and towards the affected side. Onset of familiar radiating arm pain or tingling indicates a positive test. (Photo courtesy of Diane O'Brien)

plexus. Injury may occur with shoulder dislocation, improper use of crutches, and humeral fractures. Local injury may occur from injection too close to the nerve. On physical exam, the patient may have sensory loss over a small patch on the outer shoulder as well as the inability to raise the arm.

The long thoracic nerve, the dorsal scapular nerve, and cranial nerve eleven all innervate muscles that function to rotate the shoulder blade. Each of these muscles exerts a force on one side of the triangular shoulder blade. When one of these nerves is injured, the shoulder blade is pulled in the direction of the two functioning muscles. This results in abnormal rotation or winging of the scapula. Usually, the winging itself is not painful. However, patients may notice the protruding shoulder blade in the mirror. When left unchecked, the abnormal motion may predispose patients to rotator cuff tendinopathy.

ELBOW

The elbow is a hinge joint made up of three bones, the humerus, radius, and the ulna. With the palm of the hand facing forward, the radius is located on the outside (thumb side) of the forearm. The ulna is the bone on the inside ("pinky" side) of the forearm. These two bones articulate with the large humerus. On the ulnar side, the prominence of the humerus is called the medial epicondyle. On the radial side, the prominence is called the lateral epicondyle. In the middle of these two boney protrusions rests the point of the elbow, termed the olecranon. In addition to creating a hinge on which the forearm can flex and extend, the elbow joint allows pronation and supination of the hand. Pronation occurs when the patient moves the hand palm down. Supination signifies moving the hand palm up, as would occur when carrying a bowl in the hand.

Three ligaments function to stabilize the elbow joint. The annular ligament forms a ring around the radius to hold it in place. The medial collateral ligament (MCL) is located on the inside of the forearm. The lateral collateral ligament (LCL) is located on the outside of the forearm. Sprains can occur in any of the elbow ligaments. Since the MCL provides the largest proportion of stabilization to the joint, this type of sprain can be the most detrimental. It is fairly common in young pitchers who pitch by leading with the elbow. Treatment of sprains involves relative rest, stretching, and eventual strengthening of the overlying musculature to protect the area and prevent further instability.

Elbow dislocation occurs more commonly in children than adults. Unlike shoulder dislocation, the bone frequently pops toward the back (posterior) in elbow dislocation. This can occur when the athlete tries to brace themselves from a fall by stretching out their arm. It is far less common than shoulder dislocation. Diagnosis is made when there is a posterior prominence and the patient cannot stretch out their arm. Since there are several nerves and an artery in jeopardy when this happens, careful evaluation of sensation and pulses is paramount. The dislocation can be seen on regular x-rays. Similar to shoulder dislocation, closed reduction is the mainstay of treatment. The joint is then splinted to achieve relative rest for about ten days.

In general, elbow dislocation refers to the posterior displacement of the ulna. The radius can also slip out of place. This usually occurs in toddlers when they are picked up by the arm or slip off a curb when holding the hand of an adult. The radius slips out of the annular ligament and squishes this ligament up against the ulna. Diagnosis is made when the toddler refuses to use the arm. Concurrent neurovascular injury is exceedingly rare. Treatment is much simpler than that for a true elbow dislocation. The elbow joint is manually stabilized and the wrist is pronated or supinated. Usually, the only sequela is the potential for this to happen again in the coming months. The ligaments get stronger as the child ages, and this condition is rarely seen in children over age five. The prognosis is excellent because it is a condition that the child will outgrow.

The tendons that extend the wrist run on the outside of the elbow, in the same area as the lateral collateral ligament. Lateral epicondylitis is an irritation of the tendons that attach the wrist extensors to this lateral aspect of the elbow. This is called tennis elbow because these tendons are frequently injured in amateur tennis players. Strong wrist extensors are required to resist the force of the ball against the racquet, and repetitive resistance can lead to overload of the tendon.

Golfer's elbow is the converse of lateral epicondylitis, and is called medial epicondylitis. The tendons that function to flex (or bend) the wrist start on the inside (or medial aspect) of the elbow and end at the hand. During a golf swing, there may be greater stress placed on these tendons and tendinopathy may result. Relative rest from the sport can be helpful for both tennis and golfer's elbow. In regard to golf swing mechanics, avoiding hyperextension of the elbow or hyperflexion of the wrist just prior to impact with the ball may reduce tendon inflammation or degeneration.

Little Leaguer's elbow compares to golfer's elbow in that both are tendinous injuries to the medial elbow resulting from biomechanical loads. Initially, the tendons that attach to the medial epicondyle become inflamed with the throwing motion. If this continues, it can lead to injury of the growth plate in a child or tearing off of a small piece of the medial epicondyle. When a tiny piece of bone is torn off the larger segment, this is called an avulsion fracture. For this reason, medial elbow injuries are more serious in children given the potential for bony involvement. If the growth plate is affected, this could interfere with the child's growth potential and should be carefully monitored. Injuries like these prompted the limitations on pitch counts previously mentioned.

Elbow pain in pitchers is often referred to as flexor pronator syndrome. The reason for this is that in order to increase the speed of the pitch, a great deal of stress must be put on the muscles that bend the wrist, turn the palm down, and grip the ball. These muscles are the same ones inflamed in medial epicondylitis and include the flexor carpi ulnaris, flexor carpi radialis, pronator teres, flexor digitorum profundus, flexor digitorum superficialis, and flexor pollicis longus. Tiny tears can occur in these tendons with repetitive throwing. If scar tissue forms at the area, this could decrease the ability to fully straighten the elbow. Treatment includes relative rest from pitching and physical therapy to decrease swelling, mobilize connective tissue, and improve pitching mechanics.

Since the biceps stretches from the shoulder to the elbow, it can be inflamed in either location. This muscle functions to flex (or bend) the elbow.

The biceps tendon can be felt when the athlete is bending the arm with the palm up (supination). Pain over this area indicates tendinopathy. Warmth, swelling, or redness suggests tendinitis. The treatment is the same for either condition and includes relative rest from the offending activity, ice, anti-inflammatories, and physical therapy. This injury can occur on the back of the elbow as well. The triceps muscle runs from the shoulder to the posterior elbow. Although not as common as biceps tendinopathy, triceps tendinopathy occurs with repetitive straightening of the elbow and is treated in a similar fashion.

The elbow bursa is located at the tip of the elbow, over the olecranon of the ulna. Bursitis can occur from repetitive trauma to the point of the elbow or from inflammatory arthritis. Increased fluid in the well-protected shoulder bursa rarely causes infection. However, given the superficial location of this elbow bursa, it is prone to infection when it is filled with fluid. Just like organisms grow better in a stagnant pond, bacteria can flourish in an enlarged bursal sac. Bacteria can enter the joint through abrasions in the skin.

Swelling at the point of the elbow should be evaluated for infection, especially if there is a break in the skin. Bursal infection must be treated with antibiotics. Bursal inflammation is treated similar to elbow tendinitis with ice and anti-inflammatories. The fluid can be drained off the elbow, but it often reaccumulates so this is usually done to send the fluid for diagnostics or for patient comfort rather than definitive treatment. The laboratory can run tests to assess for infection or inflammatory arthritis. Since the physical exam findings may be the same with infection or inflammation, this aids in appropriate treatment.

Arthritis is common in the hips and knees, but very rare in the elbow without prior trauma or autoimmune disease. Since most patients will remember a significant trauma, it is easy to predict whether a patient will develop this form of elbow arthritis. If a patient with no history of trauma presents with elbow arthritis, diagnostic work-up for inflammatory arthritis should be performed. Inflammatory arthridities, such as rheumatoid arthritis, may cause joint destruction in the absence of trauma. These autoimmune diseases are important to diagnose because we now have treatments that can halt the progression of disease. The earlier the treatment begins, the better the outcome for the patient. Diagnosis involves laboratory tests for inflammation in the blood and may include aspiration of the joint.

Aspiration is when a needle is inserted into the joint to draw out the fluid in the joint, called synovial fluid. This fluid is necessary to make a diagnosis. If the major finding is a large number of white blood cells, then infection is diagnosed as these cells are the infection-fighters in the body. Often, the bacteria that caused the infection can be isolated from the joint. If there are crystals, then gout or pseudogout may be diagnosed. If there are a high number of white blood cells with a characteristic appearance and no bacteria are present, then rheumatoid arthritis is suspected. The anti-ccP (anti-cyclic citrullinated peptide) blood test is gaining favor as an accurate test for rheumatoid arthritis, and joint aspiration may not be necessary unless infection is suspected. Anti-ccP antibody can be obtained from the serum to make the diagnosis.

The ulnar nerve is the reason for the pain one feels after hitting the "funny bone." This nerve courses in a groove on the medial aspect of the elbow. Due to its superficial location, it is vulnerable to injury at this area. Since the nerve feeds the ring and pinky fingers, the pain can travel down the inside of the arm to these fingers when it is struck. Loss of sensation and weakness can occur in these fingers with ulnar nerve injury. The cubital tunnel is the most common side of entrapment of the nerve. This tunnel is formed by the medial epicondyle, the olecranon, and a band of fibrous tissue that connects these two bony landmarks. If there is mechanical compression of the nerve, the nerve can be released or moved to a location where there is more space.

The anterior interosseous nerve may be injured with flexor pronator syndrome. This is the largest branch of the median nerve, which passes in front of the elbow joint. The anterior interosseous nerve feeds three muscles in the forearm: the flexor pollicis longus, the flexor digitorum profundus, and the pronator quadratus. It branches off the median nerve just after the pronator teres muscle. Although it does not innervate any of the skin, it does send braches to the wrist joint and the membrane between the two bones of the forearm. On physical exam, the patient is unable to flex the tip of the thumb, the index finger, and the middle finger, and may exhibit some difficulty with wrist pronation. Asking the patient to make an "OK" sign with the index finger and thumb will assess the affected muscles. There is no sensory loss, but there may be deep wrist pain. Anterior interosseus syndrome is more commonly seen as a manifestation of inflammation of the brachial plexus or local injury from significant trauma, but can also be seen as an entrapment neuropathy as described here and may explain the wrist pain seen with flexor pronator syndrome.

WRIST

The bones of the wrist include the radius, which articulates with the thumb, and the ulna, which attaches to the pinky side of the hand. These two larger wrist bones articulate with the many tiny bones of the hand. The scaphoid and lunate are the closest to the wrist bones. Not only can the wrist bend up and down, but it can bend side-to-side as well. When this side-to-side motion occurs toward the thumb, it is termed radial deviation. When this occurs in the opposite direction, it is called ulnar deviation.

The radius is the most commonly fractured wrist bone. This fracture can occur with a fall on the outstretched hand. Acute fracture may occur in soccer when the goalie tries to make a save and stretches out the arm while sliding sideways. A distal radius fracture has been called goalkeeper's injury for this reason. Gymnasts may get a more chronic type of fracture, called a stress fracture. This fracture occurs after repeated trauma to the bones from handstands and tumbling. Pain, swelling, and decreased range of motion on the thumb side of the wrist after trauma may indicate radial fracture. Treatment depends on the location and extent of the fracture and may include casting, surgery, or both. Stress fractures may not need to be casted, but the athlete should avoid the offending activity for at least six weeks. This type of fracture will be discussed further in the section on the foot, as these are most common in the feet and shins.

The most common tendinitis of the wrist is called DeQuervain tenosynovitis. This name comes from tendinitis and synovitis put together. Synovitis is inflammation of the lining of the joint. Pain occurs on the back side of the thumb after trauma or repetitive thumb extension as in the "thumb's up" position. The Finkelstein test is used to diagnosis this condition. The patient tucks the thumb into the palm and holds it there with the other fingers while the examiner performs ulnar deviation at the wrist. Pain in the abductor pollicis longus and extensor pollicis brevis tendons indicates a positive test. Treatment involves relative rest of the tendons by splinting the wrist. For refractory cases, steroid injection can be performed at the tendon sheath to decrease pain and inflammation.

Even without trauma, a cavity can form on the back of the wrist containing synovial fluid. A ganglion cyst is a fluid-filled sac. This feels like a bubble under the skin of the wrist and may cause pain, but is not dangerous. Since it is made of fluid, it is not a tumor. Alternatively, it is very difficult to aspirate because more fluid just fills up the cavity when it is drained. We are not really sure how the cavity occurs in the first place, but it may be related to wrist arthritis. Fluid can be removed by needle aspiration for patient comfort, but even with definitive surgical treatment, the cyst may still recur.

HAND

Given the highly specialized function of the hand, it is not surprising there are many bones connected to accomplish this. The first row of bones, closest to the wrist bones, includes the scaphoid, lunate, triquetrum, and pisiform. The trapezium, trapezoid, capitate, and hamate encompass the second row of bones. The hamate has a protrusion referred to as the hook of the hamate. The five metacarpals make up the palm of the hand, and the fourteen pha-langes make up the fingers and thumb.

Fractures of the hand can be particularly debilitating if they occur in the scaphoid. This bone can be felt on the back of the hand where the wrist turns into the thumb. Just like some of the severe shoulder and elbow fractures, this can happen when the athlete uses his or her hand to break a fall. Since the blood supply to this particular bone is tenuous, there is danger of inadequate blood supply after fracture. Fractures need vascular supply to heal. When the bone becomes injured due to decreased vascularity, we call this osteonecrosis or bone tissue death. Given this potentially devastating complication, sca-phoid fractures are monitored carefully. Serial X-rays are performed of the area even if no fracture is apparent initially. Treatment may involve casting if the bone stays in line with the other hand bones and surgery if the bone moves out of place.

Fractures of the metacarpal bones may occur during sports activity. During boxing, the metacarpals may break when striking another individual or a hard surface. Typically, this occurs in the fifth metacarpal that leads to the pinky. For this reason, a fifth metacarpal fracture is termed a boxer's fracture. The examiner can feel this bone by squeezing the palm of the hand just below the pinky. If there is swelling, tenderness, or displacement, a fracture is suspected. Treatment involves splinting and evaluation by an orthopedic hand specialist.

The fingers are able to bend at three locations due to the unique pulley sys-tem of interwoven tendons that pass through the palm. The muscles that bend the fingers are called the flexor digitorum muscles. Even though they function to move the fingers, these muscles are actually located in the medial forearm. The tendons of the flexor digitorum superficialis end at the knuckles. The flexor digitorum profundus forms tendons that course through the attachment of the flexor digitorum superficialis tendons to the ends of the fingers. These tendons can be injured during football or wrestling when one player attempts to grab another player and gets his finger stuck in the jersey. In jersey finger, the profundus tendon gets pulled off the distal phalanx and may take a tiny piece of bone with it. Diagnosis is made if the patient cannot bend the fingertip with the knuckle head steady. This injury is treated with early surgical repair.

Another problem with the flexor tendons is far more common and chronic. These tendons pass under horizontal bands connected to bone that serve as pulleys. If there is a nodule or thickening of the tendon from repetitive trauma or inflammation, this nodule may get stuck on one side of the band. If this happens with the finger bent, then the patient is unable to straighten the finger. This locking of the finger in flexion is termed trigger finger. This usually happens in athletes over age forty and may be associated with diabetes or rheumatoid arthritis. Treatment involves splinting and steroid injection or surgery for intractable cases.

The extensor tendons run on the back side of the hand, termed the dorsum. The extensor digitorum muscle functions to extend the fingers. The muscle belly is located in the lateral forearm and the tendons attach to the distal phalanx or fingertip under the nail bed. Mallet finger is when this tendon is torn from its insertion site. An avulsion fracture can occur with this type of injury as well. Diagnosis is made if the athlete cannot extend the affected digit. Splinting the finger in extension is the treatment of choice.

Carpal tunnel syndrome is often the culprit in patients who complain of numbness and tingling of the hands. This syndrome refers to compression of the median nerve at the wrist as it passes through a tunnel made up of bones and tendons. The nerve may be compressed due to local swelling, arthritis of the wrist, or thickening of the roof of the carpal tunnel formed from the transverse carpal ligament. Although this nerve lends sensation only to the thumb, index, middle, and half of the ring fingers, patients may report symptoms in all of the fingers. Typically, symptoms are worse at night and improve with shaking out the hands. Symptoms may also be exacerbated by typing on a computer. As the condition progresses, patients may notice trouble with gripping tightly or manipulating the thumb since the nerve provides motor innervation to most of the thumb muscles and one of the muscles that helps to bend the index and middle fingers.

Treatment of this very common compression neuropathy involves splinting the wrist in neutral. This refers to keeping the wrist completely in line with the hand. When the wrist is bent backward, this can put tension on an inflamed nerve and worsen the pain. When the wrist is bent forward, this can worsen the compression in the carpal tunnel. If splinting is unsuccessful, a cortisone injection or topical application of steroids may be helpful for pain. If the patient develops weakness, surgery is typically recommended. Surgery involves releasing the transverse carpal ligament. As far as surgeries go, this is a fairly successful surgery with relatively little risk.

One concern prior to surgical treatment is classification of nerve injury. Surgery is recommended for moderate to severe carpal tunnel syndrome by electrodiagnostic studies. If this abnormality is not present on the nerve studies, it may be that this is an incorrect diagnosis. A condition that is often confused with carpal tunnel syndrome is C6 radiculopathy or a pinched C6 nerve at the spine. Symptoms of C6 radiculopathy are neck pain that radiates down the outside of the arm and numbness and tingling of the thumb and index finger. Sometimes, the numbness and tingling of the thumb and index finger is so prominent in C6 radiculopathy that this condition is confused with carpal tunnel syndrome. An electrodiagnostic study is the best test to determine which diagnosis is causing the nerve pain since it looks for damage anywhere along the continuum of the nerve. A cervical spine MRI would look only for a pinched nerve at the neck; a wrist MRI would look only for compression at the carpal tunnel. Sometimes, the compression is not even visible on the wrist MRI. As such, we typically recommend electrodiagnostic studies in patients who present with numbness and tingling of the hands.

The other half of the ring finger and the pinky are innervated by the ulnar nerve. Although the most common location for entrapment of the median nerve is at the wrist, the most common location for entrapment of the ulnar nerve is actually at the elbow. Cubital tunnel syndrome was discussed in the elbow section. When the ulnar nerve gets trapped at the hand, this is usually at the Guyon's canal. This canal is formed by the pisiform and hamate bones on either side and has a ligamentous roof. Injury to the nerve at this location results in weakness of the muscles that move the pinky and the muscles that help to separate the fingers as well as sensory loss of half of the ring finger and the palmar side of the pinky finger. The back sides of these fingers are innervated by the dorsal ulnar cutaneous nerve. Since this nerve branches off the ulnar nerve prior to Guyon's canal, sensation on the back side of these fingers is maintained in ulnar neuropathy of the hand.

Compression of the ulnar nerve at Guyon's canal may occur in cyclists or triathletes from tightly gripping the handle bars of the bicycle. It can also occur in older athletes who may be using a walker to recover from hip or knee replacement. The hook of the hamate bone compresses the nerve against the handles of the bicycle or walker. The simplest treatment is the addition of padding to the handle bars or the use of cycling gloves with padding. Electrodiagnostic studies can sort out whether the compression is at the elbow or the hand. Severe cases may require surgery, but this is relatively rare.

The final nerve that innervates part of the hand is the radial nerve. The main function of this nerve is to extend the elbow and wrist. However, it does give off a superficial sensory branch that innervates the back side of the thumb. This tiny branch runs under a band of fascia called the extensor retinaculum. Numbness and tingling of the back side (or fingernail side) of the thumb are called wrist watch syndrome because the nerve can be compressed by a wrist watch or a tightly fitting wrist brace due to its superficial location. Treatment involves removing the offending agent and making sure there is no associated weakness. If there is any weakness of the wrist extensors, then the radial nerve injury is higher up than at the wrist.

SPINE

Spinal injuries receive the greatest attention among common sports injuries due to their potentially catastrophic nature. Fortunately, these injuries are becoming rare due to evolution of protective equipment and improvements in the rules of contact sports. Injury may occur when patient experiences a direct compressive force to the top of the head or a rotational force to the trunk. Given the jumping and tackling involved in football, this sport causes a significant amount of spine injuries in sports. Spear tackling, or leading with the head to tackle, is now forbidden in football for this reason. Wrestling, gymnastics, and hockey are also known for the potential to cause severe spine injuries. Protection of the spinal cord is paramount in sports as dysfunction of this large group of nerves can lead to paralysis. There are many tiny bones lined up in a column, called vertebrae, to provide this vital defense. The only part of this shield that is palpable is the spinous process, or the part of the bone that projects backward toward the skin of the back. On either side of this bony prominence, the paraspinal muscles can be felt. The ring of bone that protects the spinal cord lies deep under these muscles.

In the neck, the most prominent spinous process is that of the last cervical vertebrae. There are seven cervical vertebrae. The first cervical vertebra is unlike any of the others as it is simply a ring. This ring sits on the second cervical vertebra, which has an elongated body to make up for the lack of a vertebral body of the first. This configuration allows for more rotation at this joint. In the mid-back, there are twelve thoracic vertebrae. These bones connect to the twelve ribs that course toward the sternum, or breastbone. There are five lumbar vertebrae that make up the low back. The tailbone is made of the five bones of the sacrum. The coccyx forms the very tiny tip of this column. The main nerve that controls the function of the arms, legs, bowel, and bladder courses through the middle of this column.

Fractures can occur anywhere along this large tower of bones. In athletes, compression fractures occur when a force ruptures the anterior portion of the vertebral body (the part furthest away from where the spinal cord passes.). These are typically the best type of fractures as they do not involve disruption of the spinal ligaments and are inherently stable. This same type of fractures can occur in the thoracic spine in patients with osteoporosis. Osteoporosis signifies weak bone and a fracture can occur even with a tiny force, such as bending forward at the waist to pick something up. Most athletes rarely get osteoporosis because weight-bearing exercise prevents this condition.

Although exercise induces local bone remodeling and increased bone strength, there are important exceptions to this rule. Some athletes may have a medical condition that puts them at risk for osteoporosis. Although weight-bearing exercise is helpful in these individuals, they may still suffer from osteoporosis without other treatments to correct the underlying bone metabolism problem. If an athlete sustains a compression fracture without a trauma, the sports medicine physician must look for causes of impaired bone metabolism.

A common cause of impaired bone metabolism is estrogen deficiency. Although more estrogen is thought to increase ligamentous laxity in the younger years, less estrogen is known to unfavorably affect the bones of women as they age. Athletes with kidney problems, overactive parathyroid glands, and rheumatologic illness may also experience this poor bone health despite exercise. This issue may become increasingly important as patients are living longer and trying to exercise more with chronic illness.

There are several types of medications available to combat osteoporosis. Estrogen replacement used to be the treatment for the rapid period of bone loss that followed menopause. Now that we know that exogenous estrogen may factor in to heart disease and breast cancer, this hormone is prescribed on a more limited basis. There is a group of medicines called selective estrogen receptor modulators that works to protect bone that does not carry an increased risk of hormone-mediated cancers. In fact, these medicines were designed to fight cancer. It was discovered that they help with bone loss as well. Bisphosphonates may be a safer alternative and can be utilized in both sexes. These medicines may be taken once a week or once a month. These medicines prevent the breakdown of bone without the use of hormones or hormone receptors. They work by inhibiting cells that are charged to eat up bone. It does seem counterintuitive that the human body would have cells that break down bone, but this bone remodeling is an important process in musculoskeletal medicine. Even though bones are hard on the outside, there is a lot of exchange going on at the level of the cell. Calcium in the bloodstream is put into bone for storage. When there is not enough calcium in the bloodstream to support cellular function, it is taken out of bone. Cells that build up and break down bone function in this process along with vitamin D. For this reason, it is imperative to take calcium and vitamin D along with a bisphosphonate.

Once bone metabolism problems have been ruled out or treated, compression fracture treatment can begin. Since these fractures are inherently stable, bracing is not necessary. However, it may be utilized for patient comfort.

Patients often express a feeling of being pitched forward after this type of fracture. The reason for this is that the collapse is limited to the front portion of the bone. In an extreme case, this would be like trying to stack up a bunch of blocks shaped like squares with a block in the middle shaped like a triangle on its side. The triangle in the middle causes the blocks on top to tip forward. Braces that promote extension or arching of the back can be helpful for this feeling, but are not well-tolerated due to patient discomfort. A more realistic method involves focused strengthening of the extensor muscles of the back. That way, the patient's own muscles can be utilized to correct posture rather than a brace that they may be unlikely to wear.

Pain medications are important to incorporate to improve compliance with exercise recommendations. Formal physical therapy is best to strengthen the injured areas under supervision. Avoidance of contact sports activity for at least six weeks or until the athlete is free of pain is necessary to prevent further injury. Since the appearance of these fractures is that of a compressed front portion of the vertebrae, it is hard to assess healing with imaging. Unlike fractures in other parts of the body, there is no clear fracture line. The vertebrae will still have a partially squished appearance even when the fracture is healed. For this reason, serial imaging is not always necessary with compression fractures.

Other fractures of the spine may occur that involve a clear fracture line or even displacement of the bone. Displacement of bone is particularly concerning because of the close proximity to the spinal cord. These types of fractures usually occur after a significant bending and rotational force is applied to the spine. The severity of the fracture depends on whether any piece of bone has broken off or if the ligaments have been disrupted. Spine fractures with characteristic features have a certain nomenclature.

A Jefferson fracture denotes a fracture of the ring of the first cervical vertebra. Due to its conformation, this circular bone has to fracture in two places. (To break one part of the ossified ring, one would have to break both sides.) This type of fracture may occur when a load is applied to the top of the head. A hangman fracture is when the body of the second cervical vertebra is separated from its posterior element. An odontoid fracture is when the taller part of the body of the second cervical vertebra is detached from the rest of the body. This loose peg-like piece of bone can cause serious problems for the spinal cord. A chance fracture is a horizontal fracture of the vertebral body that occurs in the low back, often in patients who were wearing a seat belt during a car accident. These fractures are rarely associated with spinal cord injury and are not a reason to fail to wear a seat belt.

In some patients, the last lumbar vertebra may slip forward on the tail bone. This slippage is called spondylolisthesis. It usually occurs in patients who have an incompletely formed pars interarticularis, which is a small area on the back portion of the vertebrae on either side. This section of bone is right near where the vertebrae connect to each other at the facet joints. The defect in the bone may be present from birth or can occur with repetitive extension loading of the spine. If there is evidence of swelling around the defect or the appearance of a fracture line, then the latter condition is expected. This stress fracture of the spine occurs in gymnasts and wrestlers as these sports require frequent bending backward or lumbar extension. Football, rowing, and tennis also involve this motion and may predispose patients to this type of injury.

Spondylolisthesis can be diagnosed with a regular plain film because the slippage of the bones can be clearly seen on x-ray. To determine whether the associated stress fracture is present, further testing may be necessary. Bone scan demonstrates whether the injury is due to a fracture or a spinal defect from birth. MRI can show edema or soft tissue injury associated with the fracture. CT scan can clearly demonstrate the fracture line. The test ordered may depend on the time that has passed until the evaluation or the tests available at the office as all three tests may have merit in this condition.

Treatment of stress fracture of the pars interarticularis is controversial. All physicians agree that the athlete should be taken out of play until the injury is healed. The mainstay of treatment used to be bracing the athlete in a position that prevents lumbar extension for a period of three months. Unfortunately, bracing leads to atrophy of the muscles that protect the spine and few patients can be compliant with wearing a back brace for three months. Surgery is rarely required for this condition. Indications for surgery would include progression of the slippage to the point where it pinches the nerves that go down the legs.

The spinal cord connects to the brain at an important relay station for actions that we never have to think about, like breathing and maintaining wakefulness. This area is called the brainstem. The spinal cord runs from this connection, near where the spine meets the skull, to the first or second lumbar vertebrae in the low back. Then, it turns into individual nerves that run in a cluster, much like the individual hairs on a horse's tail. This section is called the cauda equina (or tail of the horse). Since these individual nerves are relatively easy to get around, spinal fluid can be obtained from this area without any lasting injury.

When a lumbar puncture or spinal tap is performed, the patient is asked to lie on his side and curl forward as if in a ball. The physician then inserts a needle between the fourth and fifth lumbar vertebrae to obtain the cerebrospinal fluid. One can palpate the area between the fourth and fifth lumbar vertebrae by putting the hands on the hips and sliding the thumbs back toward the spine. This type of procedure is done if there is suspicion for meningitis or infection around the brain or spinal cord.

Patients with meningitis complain of headaches, fever, and a stiff neck without any neck injury. Although not a common sports injury, suspicion for meningitis should exist in athletes of college age who live in close quarters and have head and neck stiffness. The goal of the spinal tap is to obtain fluid that can be analyzed for dangerous bacteria. Knowing the organism involved is important to choose the appropriate antibiotic. Another procedure done in this same area is an epidural injection. Since the goal of this injection is to deliver medicine rather than to obtain fluid, it is a more superficial and less painful procedure than a lumbar puncture. Epidural injections are done to decrease pain when a nerve is pinched in the back. Although the lumbar puncture is always done in the low back, epidural injections can be done in the neck as well since they do not go down as deep.

The spinal cord contains different pathways, called tracts, which mediate the sensation of pain, motor function, and even the position of the limb in space. Description of specific tracts is beyond the scope of this book. However, it is important to note that the spinal cord is the main nerve that controls both descending impulses from the brain and ascending impulses from the peripheral nerves. The central nervous system consists of the brain and spinal cord. The peripheral nervous system makes up all the other connections.

When the spinal cord is injured, devastating complications ensue. This type of injury usually occurs with a fracture, but may occur with a severely herniated disc or a ligamentous injury. If the spinal cord suffers a bruise, it may heal over a period of weeks. If the spinal cord is compressed and tissue death occurs, then the patient may be left paralyzed. If the injury occurs at the level of the cervical spine, this will affect the motor and sensory nerves of the arms and the legs as well as the trunk. If this injury occurs at the level of the thoracic spine, then it will affect the trunk and the legs. If the patient suffers spinal cord injury of the lumbar spine, then he or she will have weakness and sensory deficit only of the legs.

The complications of spinal cord injury go beyond the pain, muscle weakness, and inability to feel. If injury occurs in the cervical spine, the diaphragm and intercostal muscles may be affected making it difficult for the patient to breathe. Patients with spinal cord injury get pneumonia more easily for this reason. With regular physical activity, muscles help the vascular system to pump blood back to the heart. Muscle weakness in the legs can predispose patients to swelling and blood clots. The nerves that supply the bowel and bladder are made up from the bottom segments of the spinal cord. Injury at or above this level can make it difficult for the patient to urinate or defecate.

Two vertebrae converge at the facet joints and form an opening on either side termed the neural foramina. This opening houses a nerve that courses from the right or left side of the spine to the periphery. In the cervical spine, these nerves come out above the vertebrae for which they are labeled. For example, the C5 nerve courses between the C4 and the C5 vertebrae. In the thoracic and lumbar spine, the nerve courses out below the vertebrae for which it is labeled. For example, the L5 nerve exits between the L5 and the S1 vertebrae. The course of the nerves becomes particularly important when there is an obstruction in the neural foramina, such as a bone spur or a disc herniation.

After leaving the foramina, the nerve innervates different areas of muscle, skin, and even soft tissue. This is where it becomes woefully complicated. For example, the C6 nerve innervates some of the muscles that extend the wrist and bend the elbow as well as the skin on the lateral forearm and thumb. These muscles are also partially innervated by the C5 and C7 nerves. This explains how the body is evolutionarily well protected from nerve injury. When the C6 nerve is not working, the other nerves can help out and some muscle function is maintained. When a nerve is injured at the level of the nerve root, this is called radiculopathy. Patients usually call this a pinched nerve.

Radiculopathy typically results in pain that radiates from the neck or low back down the arm or leg. In cervical radiculopathy, the pain starts in the neck and goes down the arm. It is usually worse when the neck is extended toward the direction of pathology. For example, if the herniated disc is in the right neural foramina, the patient will have worsening of her symptoms when bending their head backward and to the right. The pain follows the path of the nerve. For the C6 nerve, the pain often radiates down the outside of the arm into the thumb and/or index finger.

Just as in the cervical spine, radiculopathy symptoms in the lumbar spine depend on the path of the nerve. The most common nerves to get pinched are the L5 or S1 nerve roots, located just above the tailbone. Pain from the L5 nerve is typically down the side of the leg into the top of the foot. Pain in the S1 nerve goes down the back of the leg into the bottom of the foot. Often, patients will call this type of pain sciatica. The sciatic nerve is actually made up of the L4, L5, S1, and S2 nerve roots. It begins where these nerves form a large cord in the buttock. Symptoms are usually worsened by raising the leg from a supine position. This test is called the straight leg test. It augments pain by putting tension on the nerve as it exits the spine and courses down the back or side of the leg. It is considered positive when the pain is in the leg rather than in the back.

Other less common areas of pinched nerves in the low back are the L1 through L4 nerve roots. The L1 nerve root innervates the groin area. The L2 nerve root innervates the skin of the mid-thigh. The L3 nerve root innervates the knee and may be confused with anterior knee problems. The L4 nerve root innervates the inside part of the shin and arch of the foot. Pinching of any of the L2 through L4 nerve roots may result in pain when the femoral nerve is stretched. With the patient lying face-down, the examiner bends the affected knee and pulls the leg up toward the ceiling. Anterior thigh pain with this test, called the femoral nerve stretch test, suggests a pinched nerve at one of these levels. A decreased knee reflex on the side of the pain also suggests a pinched nerve at the L2, L3, or L4 level. Unfortunately, impingement at any of these levels may give a positive test. Imaging is often needed to sort out the exact level due to overlapping innervation and lack of a specific test for each nerve.

Treatment involves anti-inflammatories to decrease the pain and physical therapy to strengthen the back muscles and prevent scarring of the nerve. Corticosteroids are the strongest anti-inflammatory that we have in our armentarium. In an epidural injection, steroids are injected at the area of the injured nerve to decrease swelling and pain. Steroids do not make the herniated disc go away, but they can help with the associated inflammatory reaction that occurs as a result of the herniation.

Disc injuries are unique to the spine. In between each vertebra, there lays a cushion made of shock absorbent material. The inside portion of the disc is made of a jelly-like substance called the nucleus pulposis. The outside portion is made from a fibrous ring of tissue called the annulus fibrosis. When a tear in the annulus fibrosis occurs, a small amount of jelly can leak out and irritate the spinal fluid or the nerves. This is called an annular tear and may cause localized back pain. There are tiny nerves that feed the annulus that carry this signal back to the brain. Disc pain is typically worse with coughing or sneezing.

If the nucleus pulposus pushes out of a tear in the annulus fibrosis, this is called a herniated disc. The biggest concern with a herniated disc is that it pushes on the nerve, as in radiculopathy. There are three types of herniated discs: protrusion, extrusion, and sequestration. In protrusion or prolapse, the disc pushes out past the annulus fibrosis. This is the mildest form of disc herniation. In extrusion, the disc material pushes out and drips over, forming the appearance of a teardrop on MRI. In sequestration, the portion of disc that pushed out is separated from the parent disc. This separation makes it harder for this type of herniation to heal. Sometimes, the disc fragment needs to be surgically repaired.

In general, treatment of disc herniation is symptomatic. Physical therapy, medications, and epidural injections are the usual conservative treatments. Bed rest beyond three days is discouraged. Walking increases blood flow to the spine, and should be performed as tolerated. About 75 percent of patients improve in six to twelve months without surgical intervention. If the patient has leg weakness or urinary retention, surgical consultation is necessary.

Unfortunately, both the epidural injections and the surgery work better for leg pain than back pain. Numbness may or may not improve with these measures. Urinary retention may be an indication of cauda equine syndrome or compression of the nerves that feed the bowel, bladder, and legs. Although rare, cauda equina syndrome is a surgical emergency. Patients with this syndrome typically lose sensation in their genital area and have trouble urinating. Urinary or fecal frequency or incontinence may also be seen. Treatment involves surgical decompression.

Since the discs are the shock absorbers of the spine, activities that require shock absorption like running or jumping are generally avoided for the first six weeks. Walking and stretching is encouraged. Often, the spinal muscles will spasm to protect the injured area, and these muscles need to be stretched or massaged to feel better. Activating the antagonist muscle groups may also encourage relaxation of the muscles over the disc herniation. Under the direction of a physical therapist, strength training of the back muscles should be performed. Since the body is like a cylinder, strengthening of the back muscles must occur in conjunction with strengthening of the abdominal muscles to achieve optimal results.

Disc herniation is commonly confused with disc bulge. These are two very different problems. A disc herniation is more of an acute injury, and a disc bulge is a manifestation of prior disc injury or the loss of water in the disc due to age-related changes. Many people without pain have disc bulges found incidentally on MRI. This makes them harder to treat. Most doctors believe that disc bulges are the beginnings of spine arthritis and do not need any treatment if there is no pain associated with them.

If pain is associated with a disc bulge, the problem becomes more complicated. We can carefully visualize all of the structures in the spine on MRI, but we cannot determine which structure is causing the pain. Some studies have tried to improve our understanding of pain generators in the spine by injecting anesthetic and/ or steroid into these structures and monitoring for pain relief. In general, pain that radiates down the arm or leg associated with numbness and tingling tends to respond best to injection around the nerve. Pain that is localized to the neck or back and is worse with looking at the ceiling or arching the low back responds best to facet injection or injection at the joint. Pain in the muscle may respond to local injection, massage, or spinal manipulation.

Despite the severity of the patient's pain, the most common cause of back pain is not a pinched nerve or a disc herniation. The most common cause of low back pain is lumbar strain. This type of injury is frequently seen in the weight room after practice, especially in the teenage years. There are multiple layers of muscles around the spine. Closest to the bones, there are tiny muscles that run between two vertebrae. On top of these muscles, there are larger muscles that span even more vertebrae. All of the muscles that cover the bones of the spine function to extend the spine or arch the back. When picking up heavy weights off the ground, it is easy to imagine that one might strain these muscles that resist this motion. The act of being pushed backward, which occurs frequently in football and hockey, can also strain the lumbar extensors. Treatment involves a brief period of rest from lifting. Walking is always permitted during this time period as it is a safe and healthy exercise for the back. If there is any leg pain or the back pain persists beyond four to six weeks, imaging may be necessary to make sure there is no associated injury.

To successfully return to sport after lumbar strain injury, physical therapy can be extremely helpful. Initially, physical therapy will focus on stretching the low back extensors, the hip extensors, and the hip rotators. With back problems it is important to stretch out the hips because muscles from both the hip and the back can affect the tilt of the pelvis. If the pelvis tilts too much toward one of these groups of muscles, this can worsen muscle strain. Also, the psoas muscle joins with the iliacus muscle in the pelvis to flex the hip. Because the psoas attaches to the sides of the vertebrae in the low back, hip motion may exacerbate lumbar strain. This can occur in soccer players when they kick the ball. Hip flexion against the resistance of the soccer ball may exacerbate back pain due to the attachments of the iliopsoas muscle. Stretching of the hip flexors may be an important component of return to play in soccer.

After stretching out the spasm, strengthening is important to protect the injured area. The strengthening phase of rehabilitation should affect not only the lumbar extensors, but also the abdominal musculature. The human body is shaped like a cylinder. It is important to strengthen both sides of the cylinder to achieve the best outcome. For this reason, pilates and yoga have come into favor for athletes in all sports. There really is medical evidence behind the old joke of the football player who signs up for ballet class to improve his game.

Back pain is so common that there are many professionals who deal with this problem. Spinal manipulation can be effective whether performed by a chiropractor, physical therapist, or doctor of osteopathy. A patient may get relief from seeing the massage therapist or the acupuncturist. These modalities are very difficult to study because studies are set up with an experimental group and a control group. For example, the experimental group will get the real medicine and the control group gets a fake pill called a placebo. Since we have no way to give fake acupuncture or massage, it is difficult to determine their efficacy. There are no hard data to say which treatment is better. Regardless, these treatments have very little risk associated with them and they often decrease pain. The right answer is whatever treatment is able to provide the most relief for the patient. Currently, insurance companies may give a discount for acupuncture or chiropractic treatment, but do not fully cover these services. Unfortunately, cost becomes another important factor in the choice for treatment of back pain.

The first step is diagnosis. Once the doctor has determined there is no underlying disc herniation or nerve injury, pain control is recommended. The pain control phase may include spinal manipulation, massage, acupuncture, ice, or heat. In general, ice is best for the first forty-eight hours. Ice is the treatment for inflammation, and heat is the treatment for spasm. Since most patients experience both phenomena, I usually recommend heat before activity to loosen up the muscle and ice after to help decrease the local inflammatory reaction. Topical medications can also be helpful. These over-the-counter medications usually include menthol and a derivative of aspirin. They should be applied according to the package instructions, and the skin should not be occluded after application.

Medications used to treat back pain include anti-inflammatories, nerve pain medications, and muscle relaxants. Anti-inflammatories work by decreasing the cells that mediate pain and are more helpful in the first two weeks of pain or injury. Side effects include stomach upset and worsening of pre-existing kidney problems. Nerve pain medications include gabapentin and pregabalin. These medications were initially used to treat seizures until we learned that they could be helpful for nerve pain. Side effects include fatigue, swelling, and mood changes in a small number of patients. The category of muscle relaxants encompasses medications like cyclobenzaprine and tizanidine. These medicines may cause far more fatigue than nerve pain medications because they work on the brain to relax the muscles. Patients should not drive on these medications, and they need to be taken only at night to help with sleep. In a small number of patients, liver problems have been reported.

Lumbar stenosis refers to a narrowing of the holes where the nerves live. Central stenosis means narrowing of the main middle hole through which the spinal cord and cauda equina pass. This hole should have about a one-centimeter diameter to accommodate the nerves. Foraminal stenosis means narrowing of the passageway for the individual nerve roots on the sides of the spine. These holes can become acutely narrowed due to a disc herniation as previously mentioned. More commonly, they become narrow over time due to the degenerative changes that are so common in the spine.

Typically, there is not one single structure that causes the lumbar stenosis. Degeneration of the discs brings the bones closer together and the disc may sag into the spinal canal. Osteoarthritis can occur at the facet joints. Bone spurs can poke into the spinal canal. Ligaments can develop fibrosis or calcifications. It is the combination of all of these degenerative changes that yields stenosis. Fortunately, this process takes time. This condition is rarely seen in athletes under the age of sixty-five. There is one exception to this rule. Some patients are born with a spinal canal that is too small to start with. In these patients, a little bit of arthritis goes a long way to narrow the canal.

Lumbar stenosis usually causes pain in the back and down one or both legs that is worse with walking. The pain is often relieved with bending forward. The reason for this is that the holes become smaller when the back is arched. Lumbar flexion or bending forward at the waist allows more room in the area where the nerves pass. This type of pain is called neurogenic claudication.

Pain down the legs in older athletes can also be a result of vascular claudication. This is when the legs hurt because they are not getting adequate blood flow. Both types of pain typically get worse with walking. However, vascular claudication tends to get better more quickly with rest than neurogenic claudication. Also, vascular claudication tends to be worse when going uphill than flat surfaces. Neurogenic claudication may improve slightly when going uphill because bending forward at the waist is required to walk uphill.

If we are unable to determine the problem from the patient's history, there are some helpful clues on physical exam. In patients with vascular claudication, pulses in the feet are decreased or may not be palpable. The typical pattern of hair growth is reduced due to reduced blood supply. There may be swelling of the lower limbs or increased skin pigmentation due to pooling of blood. Patients with isolated neurogenic claudication do not typically have these findings, but often have decreased pin prick sensation of the lower limbs. Patients with signs of both neurogenic and vascular claudication require further testing. A lumbar MRI can determine whether there is lumbar stenosis. Doppler studies of the vasculature can measure the flow of blood. Ankle–brachial indices are the study of choice at most institutions to quantify lumbar stenosis.

The ankle–brachial index is a ratio of the blood flow in the legs compared to the arms. Blood pressure is taken in the leg and arm at rest. If the ankle blood pressure is equal to the brachial or arm blood pressure, then the measurement is 1.0, which is normal. If the ratio is 0.8, then vascular claudication is present. If the ratio is even lower, the patient may have vascular problems at rest. Usually, an ankle–brachial index of 0.5 or below requires surgical intervention. Initial treatment of vascular claudication is usually compression stockings and medications that help decrease the swelling. If the blood flow becomes compromised, then a graft is placed at the area of compromise so the blood can flow freely again.

Once the source of leg pain is determined to be neurogenic claudication from lumbar stenosis, treatment can begin. Conservative treatment is similar to that for a pinched nerve and includes physical therapy, medication management, and epidural steroid injections. Definitive treatment of lumbar stenosis is decompression surgery.

Unlike a disc herniation, which can resorb on its own, the degenerative changes from lumbar stenosis do not go away. Remarkably, not all patients experience worsening pain with worsening stenosis. Sometimes, the bone spurs grow together and fuse the joint surfaces. Patients with less joint motion due to fusion may have less pain. Some patients just get better for reasons we cannot explain. Generally, surgery is recommended if the the leg pain becomes too much to bear, if there is leg weakness, or if the bowel or bladder is affected.

HIP

Knute Rockne advised that "a bruised hip should be treated and protected much the same as a bruised shoulder. Form a cup over the injured part." Protecting the hip with a cup would work well for injuries to the greater trochanter, the bony projection on the lateral aspect of femur, but it would be very unsuccessful to protect the true hip joint. The hip is certainly a joint that we have learned much more about since Rockne suggested this treatment in the 1930s.

Unlike the shoulder, the hip is a ball inside a socket. It is well situated and usually has to break to dislocate. The hip joint consists of the femur (thigh bone) and its socket (the acetabulum). The acetabulum is part of the pelvis. Just to make it confusing, the bones of the pelvis have different names depending on their location. The ischium is the part of the pelvis that you sit on, and the ilium is the part that makes up the sides of the pelvis. The ischium is that bony prominence that gives the patient sore buttocks when riding a bike or motorcycle. The crests of the ilium are where patients would put their hands when told to put their hands on their hips. The sacrum, otherwise known as the tailbone, forms the back of the pelvis.

The femur contains the ball part of the hip joint and is the longest bone in the body. There are two outpouchings of bone on the femur that become important in assessing soft tissue injury. The greater trochanter, as mentioned above, is the prominence on the lateral aspect of the femur. This prominence is palpable on the outside of the leg below the iliac crest. It is the part of the hip the patient lies on when in a side-lying position. The lesser trochanter cannot be palpated due to its smaller size and deeper location in the medial thigh.

The acetabulum is made from the bones of the pelvis. Since the bones of the pelvis are such strong bones, it requires a significant force for them to fracture. When this occurs, the pelvis will fracture in two places. Imagine the pelvis as a pretzel; in order to break in one place, it must break in another. Diagnosis involves finding all of the potential pelvic fractures. Treatment involves pain control, activity restriction, and gradual return to hip exercises to strengthen the overlying soft tissues.

There is one exception to the rule that where there is one pelvic fracture, there must be another. Isolated fractures may occur if the fracture is of the insufficiency or stress fracture type. This type of fracture is not from trauma, but from a weakness in the bone. The weakness can be due to a metabolic bone disease or to simply not getting enough calcium and vitamin D, which are the building blocks of bone. When seen in isolation or without trauma, a pelvic fracture will usually be of this type. Treatment of this type of fracture often requires a visit to the endocrinologist (hormone specialist) or rheumatologist (specialist in inflammatory diseases) in addition to the usual fracture management.

Similar to the scaphoid bone in the hand, the hip is one of the areas in the body that is prone to avascular necrosis due to a tenuous blood supply after traumatic injury. Bone cells receive nutrients from the blood constantly. Avascular necrosis or osteonecrosis refers to death of bone cells when this process halts. This disorder not only may occur with trauma, but also can occur spontaneously with a host of medical problems that may interfere with vascular nutrient delivery.

Possible etiologies of avascular necrosis include alcohol abuse, sickle cell anemia, lupus, HIV infection, or organ transplantation. The exact mechanism of osteonecrosis is unclear in these diseases, but overall the pathology is related to metabolic dysfunction of the bone cells. Without nutrients, the bone loses its mineral content. Since the minerals make up the framework of bone, the bone structure collapses in their absence. Use of certain medical therapies has also been implicated in bone cell death. These therapies include radiation treatment, bisphosponate use in patients with cancer, and long-term glucocorticoid use.

Avascular necrosis presents in a similar fashion to hip osteoarthritis. Patients typically complain of groin pain. The pain is worse with walking and may be associated with morning stiffness. The patient may have difficulty bending his or her hip to rise from a chair. Not only are symptoms similar to those of osteoarthritis, but appearance on radiographs is similar as well. As the condition progresses, there may be a dark line inside the bone with the same shape as the ball of the femur called *a crescent sign*. Although it may show up on radiographs or bone scan, earliest diagnosis of osteonecrosis is typically made by MRI as this is the most sensitive test. Treatment involves hip resurfacing or replacement, especially if suspected collapse of bone is imminent.

Although the hip joint is designed for weight-bearing and the shoulder joint is designed for a large arc of motion, both joints have a labrum. Just like in the shoulder, the labrum of the hip is a ring of fibrocartilage that encircles the joint. Similar to the shoulder, the hint of a labral tear may be seen on MRI, but cannot be seen on X-ray. Often, the labrum is not fully visualized on MRI. The best test to visualize the labrum is an MRI after dye has been injected into the joint, called an MR arthrogram. The dye outlines the joint and makes a tear in the labrum easier to see.

The challenging part is what to do after a labral tear is diagnosed. The outside part of the labrum has a blood supply and may heal on its own. Surgical consultation should be obtained if there is clicking or locking of the hip joint or the tear includes more than the outer rim. Typically, arthroscopic surgery is done to repair the labrum, but each case is carefully evaluated clinically as we are still learning the best ways to treat this. If the labral tear is associated with osteoarthritis, it may be very difficult to tell which problem is causing the hip pain.

The most common sports injury of the hip is muscle strain. The muscle involved depends on the location of the pain. When an athlete complains of a pulled groin, they are referring to an adductor strain. The adductor group of muscles is on the inside of the thigh and includes the gracilis (closest to the skin), adductor magnus, adductor longus, adductor brevis, and pectineus (closest to the pelvic bones). These muscles function to bring the thighs closer together, the action that would occur if a patient were trying to squeeze a tennis ball between his or her knees. The quadriceps in the front of the thigh and the hamstrings in the back of the thigh can also suffer from strain. Usually, pain from muscle strain will gradually subside over a few weeks with discontinuation of the offending activity. If bruising is present or bulge is seen under the skin, the patient should be evaluated by a physician as this may be a sign of tearing of the muscle.

When patients complain of hip pain, an important question is whether the pain is in the front, the side, or the back of the hip. Usually, hip joint problems result in inguinal, or groin pain. Pain in the side of the hip often indicates a problem with the trochanteric bursa, iliotibial band, or hip rotators. When the pain is in the buttock, it is more likely from a spine problem or a muscle problem than true hip joint pathology. Since the hip is such a difficult joint to palpate, physicians will often base their diagnostic impression on hip range of motion maneuvers. Inguinal pain with internal rotation of the hip suggests hip joint pathology. Tenderness over the lateral hip suggests greater trochanteric bursitis or iliotibial band syndrome. Buttock pain with resisted external rotation of the hip on exam suggests spine or gluteal muscle pathology.

Collisions in contact sports may result in a hip pointer, a commonly used term referring to an injury over the iliac crest (top part of the ilium). The injury can be a bone contusion with or without an avulsion fracture. A bone contusion is a collection of fluid and blood that forms in an area of bone injury. An avulsion fracture means that a piece of the bone is pulled off of the iliac crest, usually by a tendon. Since tendons are the attachment of muscles to bones, muscles potentially involved include the sartorius, tensor fascia lata, rectus femoris, and abdominal obliques because they attach at this location.

Tendinopathy can occur in many places around the hip joint. The iliopsoas muscle originates on the sides of the lumbar vertebrae and ends on the inside prominence of the femur called the lesser trochanter. Tendinopathy of this muscle results in groin pain with resisted hip flexion. Hamstring tendinopathy presents as pain localized to the ischium in the buttocks that worsens with resisted knee flexion and may radiate to the back of the knee if the muscles in the back of the thigh are stretched. The iliotibial band originates on the iliac crest and stretches over the greater trochanter to insert on the outside of the knee. Tendinopathy of the iliotibial band may cause pain down the outside of the thigh that radiates to the outside of the knee when one leg is stretched across the other.

Classically, tendinopathy of the gluteal musculature will result in buttock pain or lateral hip pain. The gluteus medius muscle, which helps the athlete lift the leg when lying on the side or spread the legs apart, inserts on the greater trochanter. As mentioned previously, the greater trochanter is a bony prominence of the femur present at the widest part of the hips. Pain in this area may indicate gluteus medius tendinopathy, iliotibial band syndrome, or greater trochanteric bursitis. Of note, pain in this area does not always signify a hip problem. The L5 nerve root from the spine innervates the side of the leg in the same area as the iliotibial band. One of the ways we sort out these two diagnoses is to ask the patient if the pain goes below the knee or is associated with numbness and tingling. Since the iliotibial band does not go below the knee, injury at this area does not usually result in calf pain. Numbness and tingling are highly suggestive of nerve pain and do not usually occur in a syndrome isolated to the muscle.

Iliotibial band syndrome signifies a tightness of this muscle that results in lateral hip pain. It is common in runners who do not stretch after working out. Greater trochanteric bursitis is inflammation of the fluid-filled sac that covers the greater trochanteric bursa. Since these three problems all cause lateral hip pain, they are often referred to as greater trochanteric pain syndrome. Treatment involves pain relief, stretching of the iliotibial band and hip rotators, and eventual progression to strengthening of the hip rotators. Bursitis tends to recur if underlying muscle imbalances are not treated.

Although there are many tendons that could potentially result in a tendinitis at the hip, there are really only three areas where bursitis occurs. We commonly refer to the greater trochanteric bursa as one single fluid-filled sac. However, there are really two to three fluid-filled sacs in this area to cushion the bony prominence and allow the tendons of the hip rotators to glide smoothly. Typically, injection of the area with corticosteroids provides relief regardless of which bursa is entered. This type of bursitis is easily seen on MRI of the hip.

The deep hip bursa is the iliopsoas bursa. This bursa is buried under significant soft tissue, and can only be accessed with an injection done under x-ray guidance. Since this type of bursitis is hard to visualize on MRI, the diagnosis is made on clinical exam. If the patient had no trauma to the iliopsoas muscle and has pain with hip hyperflexion, this is suggestive of iliopsoas bursitis. The diagnosis is confirmed if the patient gets relief with injection of the bursa.

Bursitis of the posterior hip frequently occurs in cyclists or triathletes. The ischial bursa lies over the ischium and adjacent to the tendons of the hamstring muscles. It is more prominent when seated than when standing. In standing, the large superficial muscle that extends the thigh, called the gluteus maximus, coves the prominence. When biking, the area comes in contact with the bike seat. Prolonged sitting on a bike, especially over bumpy terrain, can irritate this area. Care must be taken when injecting this bursa as the sciatic nerve lies just to the outside of the bony prominence. I usually recommend relative rest, local ice treatments, and hamstring stretching prior to consideration of injection given the slightly increased risk in this area.

Another common soft tissue condition of the hip that affects athletes is snapping hip. There are two areas where snapping may occur. The iliotibial band is a band of muscle and fascia that begins on the iliac crest and bows over the greater trochanter to end on the lateral condyle of the tibia. This thin strap-like muscle helps to flex and rotate the hip. Given its small diameter, it contributes little to these actions. It may snap over the large greater trochanter. This can be felt on exam if the patient crosses one leg over the other and turns the foot inward and outward while maintaining a straight leg.

Snapping of the iliopsoas muscle is more difficult to feel on exam. The iliopsoas muscle is actually formed from two separate muscles that function together. The psoas major starts on the front and sides of the lumbar vertebrae and joins with the iliacus to insert on and below the lesser trochanter of the femur. The iliacus starts on the inside of the ilium and joins with the psoas deep in the pelvis. The common tendon is thought to snap over the lesser trochanter or the pectineal eminence. This may be felt in the groin if the patient tries to straighten the hip from a bent position.

Snapping is typically not dangerous to the patient. In fact, it is often present in dancers and may be a sign of increased flexibility. A tendon is prone to the snapping when it is too stretched or loose. Although it is very easy to treat tight muscles with stretching, it is much more difficult to treat loose tendons or instability. If the snapping is accompanied by severe pain, imaging may be helpful to rule out associated avulsion fracture or labral tear. Treatment involves avoiding the offending activity. For example, patients with iliopsoas tendon snapping should avoid biking. The iliopsoas is a strong hip flexor and biking requires repetitive hip flexion. Strengthening of the hip rotators and gluteal muscles may also be helpful to protect the overstretched tendons.

Diagnostic imaging becomes far more important in the hip due to its deep location and our lack of adequate physical exam maneuvers. Most of these maneuvers can isolate the problem to an area of the hip, but not to a specific structure. If the patient has primarily anterior or inguinal pain, had a trauma, or is greater than sixty-five years of age, hip radiographs are indicated to look for bone pathology or arthritis. If the patient has buttock pain and numbness and tingling, a lumbar spine MRI would be the best test to check the nerves as they exit the spine. Most patients fall between these two categories. Frequently, patients complain of a groin pain that started in the buttock or a buttock pain that started in the groin. Even after hip exam, there can be some confusion as to the area of pathology given the deep location of the joint and the many large muscles that pass through the pelvis.

Once the cause of hip pain is determined, physical therapy can be initiated. Most soft tissue injuries improve with stretching and strengthening. If the pain persists beyond two months, an MRI may be helpful to further target treatment. MRI of the lumbar spine should be performed if the pain is in the posterior hip. An MRI of the hip should be performed if the pain is in the anterior or the lateral hip as only bone pathology can be viewed on radiographs. For refractory pain, advanced imaging is necessary to find a potential target for intervention and make sure there is no underlying abnormality perpetuating the muscle dysfunction. Potential problems that may show up on MRI that would not show up on radiographs would be a stress fracture, early osteoarthritis, labral tear, or avascular necrosis.

If the patient is unable to tolerate physical therapy due to the pain and there is no avascular necrosis or underlying fracture, a cortisone injection may be helpful to relieve the pain. Patients with fractures should not have a cortisone injection because this can delay healing. For pain in the lateral hip, a cortisone injection into the greater trochanteric bursa is performed. This type of injection can be done in the regular clinic office with a needle filled with cortisone and anesthetic. For treatment of deep inguinal pain associated with hip joint problems on imaging, an injection deep in the hip joint is done. This type of injection must be done under fluoroscopic, or X-ray, guidance as it is important to get the medicine in the correct area.

Steroid and anesthetic injection may provide relief if the pain is from an iliopsoas bursitis, hip osteoarthritis, or labral tear. Of note, glucocorticoids are the same medicine as "cortisone" or "steroid." With less than four steroid injections per year, avascular necrosis is unlikely to occur. Most patients with avascular necrosis from glucocorticoids have taken oral steroids for years. This is difficult to study as patients on steroids may have other diagnoses that predispose them to avascular necrosis. In general, oral steroid doses of 20 milligrams or more of prednisone are thought to put patients at increased risk.

As the population ages, there are more athletes with hip osteoarthritis. This condition is a very common cause of disability in the general population as well as in athletes. Traumatic injury is associated with arthritis in one hip. Remarkably, arthritis in both hips may actually be associated with inactivity. Although genetics certainly plays a role, inactivity leads to obesity. Patients who carry more weight tend to have more arthritis in weight-bearing joints like the hip and the knee. We used to caution patients with arthritis about too much exercise. Now, we recommend exercise as a treatment for osteoarthritis.

Pain in the groin is usually the first symptom of osteoarthritis of the hip. The pain is typically associated with stiffness. Patients often complain of difficulty bending the hip, as might occur in the twisting motion of golf. On physical exam, the complaint of groin pain when the examiner internally rotates the patient's hip suggests hip pathology. Decreased internal range of motion on hip exam is usually the first positive diagnostic sign for hip osteoarthritis. Later, range of motion may decrease in hip flexion and external rotation. As arthritis progresses, patients may develop a limp. Trendelenburg sign is when the gluteus medius becomes weak and the pelvis tilts with ambulation. This sign is commonly seen in patients with hip osteoarthritis due to changes in the joint space and weakness of the hip rotators that may accompany arthritis.

At minimum, radiographs are necessary to assess for loss of joint space, brightening of the bone at the joint interface from rubbing, and the formation of cysts that may occur with osteoarthritis. If these features are present in a young patient with no known trauma, MRI may be necessary to check for avascular necrosis as a cause of the hip joint collapse. Blood labs may be helpful to look for causes of autoimmune disease. It is important to make sure there is no associated systemic illness in a patient who has unexplainable arthritis. Unfortunately, osteoarthritis is incredibly common and may affect some patients earlier in life for reasons we cannot yet explain.

Initially, treatment of hip osteoarthritis involves anti-inflammatory medication and physical therapy. The goal of physical therapy is to strengthen the gluteal muscles that help to stabilize the hip joint. One of my mentors likes to joke that the gluteus maximus sticks out and takes all the credit. The maximus is that large muscle closest to the surface of the buttocks that functions to extend the joint. Although this muscle is necessary to help you return to standing when bent over, it is not particularly helpful in stabilizing the hip joint. The key muscle is under the maximus.

The gluteus medius and minimus lie under the gluteus maximus and act to abduct the hip. Hip abduction refers to spreading the legs apart. While walking, these muscles function as key stabilizers to keep the pelvis level. When the weight-bearing surface of the hip wears away, the forces at this joint may change. One way to protect the joint is to strengthen the muscles that hold the pelvis level in ambulation. These muscles can be strengthened in side-lying by lifting the upper leg toward the sky with the knee facing forward. Once this activity can be performed pain-free, a circular ankle weight can be added to raise the level of difficulty. If the athlete is unable to perform leg lifts in side-lying, another option is to stand close to a wall and press the side of the foot into the wall with the toes facing forward (long axis of the foot parallel to the wall). A slight burn deep in the buttocks might be felt after these exercises.

When exercise no longer helps for the pain, the hip joint may be too worn to function adequately. If the patient has trouble climbing stairs or simply walking from hip arthritis, the orthopedic surgeon will usually recommend hip replacement. Hip replacement surgery is typically done with metal, plastic, or ceramic parts. Similar to the shoulder, replacement of only the ball part of the joint is called a partial hip replacement and the insertion of both a new ball and a new socket is called a total hip replacement. The type of procedure and material used depends on the extent of the arthritis and the activity level of the patient.

After surgery, rehabilitation plays a pivotal role in regaining function and returning to athletic activity. Often, patients will use a cane or a walker until they feel steady with the new joint. Although this occurs in only 2 percent to 4 percent of patients, a potential problem after hip replacement is dislocation of the new joint. To prevent this problem, the physical therapist instructs the patient in ways to prevent dislocation, commonly referred to in the hospital as hip precautions. If the hip was inserted through the back side of the patient's hip, the concern is that the hip could dislocate posteriorly. To prevent this, patients are instructed to sit in chairs or toilets with a special booster seat that will not allow the hips to bend more than 90 degrees. Once patients have mastered the hip precautions, they can move on to climbing stairs and hip-strengthening exercises.

Another uncommon complication of joint replacement is infection. Although rare, this can be devastating when it occurs. Bacteria grow favorably in foreign bodies and in areas of stagnant fluid or swelling. Unfortunately, both of these circumstances are present in hip replacement. As long as the infection is caught early, the replacement joint can usually be washed out and the patient treated with antibiotics. If the infection occurs later on, removal of the device and more aggressive antibiotic treatment may be necessary. Some patients require antibiotic prophylaxis prior to dental procedures for a period after hip replacement to prevent infection. These recommendations have changed over the years and should be reviewed with the surgeon prior to dental work.

Nerve injury may occur after hip replacement. Often, this is from surgical positioning or prolonged bed rest and resolves spontaneously when the patient is up and moving again. Typically, patients have an exacerbation of pain that radiates down the back or side of the leg. This is particularly common in patients who have concurrent spine problems. If weakness is present, physician evaluation is essential. The sciatic nerve is the one most commonly irritated after hip replacement. Other nerves that may be injured include the femoral and obturator nerves. The femoral nerve runs down the front of the leg and the obturator nerve courses through the inside of the thigh.

Nearly one-fourth of patients experience leg length discrepancy after hip replacement. A number of factors may account for the feeling that one leg is longer than the other. The most common contributor to this problem is tightening of the hip rotators. In this case as in many of the hip joint problems, the gluteus medius and minimus are central to the issue. Other hip rotators are the piriformis, the gemelli, and the quadratus femoris. Tightening or spasm in any of these muscles could result in the feeling that one leg is shorter than the other. One exam, leg length is typically measured from the anterior superior iliac spine (on the front of the iliac crest) to the medial malleolus on the inside of the ankle. If there is a difference of more than one inch from side-to-side, then a lift in the shoe might be recommended. Stretching exercises are usually tried before or in conjunction with a heel lift to treat the underlying cause of the problem.

Pain in the hip area can also be from pathology outside the hip. Radiating pain associated with numbness and tingling is typical of nerve pain. The sciatic nerve is the largest nerve in the sacral plexus and in the human body. Sciatica refers to pain in the distribution of this nerve and is a common condition in athletes over fifty years of age. Since the nerve runs down the buttock and side of the leg into the foot, this is the distribution of pain. The patient will feel worsening of this pain when the examiner lifts the affected leg upward with the patient lying on his or her back. The sciatic nerve is made up of lower lumbar and upper sacral nerve roots that exit the neural foramina on either side of the spine and form a large trunk in the buttock. This large trunk travels under a pear-shaped muscle in the buttock called the piriformis.

Prior to MRI, we used to think sciatica was due to piriformis syndrome. In piriformis syndrome, the sciatic nerve gets compressed by the muscle of the same name. From cadaveric studies, we have learned that very few patients actually have a piriformis muscle that obstructs the course of the nerve. A possible scenario is that the muscle develops swelling or spasm, which irritates the nerve. Although this may be the case, many of the patients previously diagnosed with piriformis syndrome have narrowing in the lumbar spine around the L5 or S1 nerve root on MRI. If there is obstruction of the nerve at the level of the spine, it is difficult to argue for isolated piriformis syndrome. The piriformis muscle is innervated by the lower sacral roots. It could spasm from pinching of the S1 nerve around the spine. Regardless of the cause, piriformis spasm often accompanies sciatica. Treatment involves avoiding the potential cause of nerve irritation, stretching of the piriformis muscle and the other hip rotators, hamstring stretching, and pain control with anti-inflammatories, muscle relaxants, or nerve pain medications.

Sciatica could explain posterior hip pain or radiating leg pain that goes down the back or side of the leg. It does not cause anterior hip pain. For patients with nerve pain that radiates down the front of the leg, diagnostic possibilities include high lumbar radiculopathy, lateral femoral cutaneous neuropathy, and femoral neuropathy. High lumbar radiculopathy refers to a pinched nerve at either the L1 or L2 levels. The L1 nerve innervates the groin area. The L2 nerve innervates the skin of the mid-thigh as well as lends partial innervation to muscles that help bend and rotate the hip. Either type of pinched nerve may give a sensory deficit in the anterior thigh. Impingement of the L2 nerve may also exhibit weakness of the hip flexors or a slightly decreased reflex at the knee. The best way to diagnose a lumbar radiculopathy is with an MRI of the low back.

The lateral femoral cutaneous nerve provides sensory input for the outside, or lateral aspect, of the thigh. Impingement of this nerve is also called meralgia paresthetica. This condition is often a diagnosis of exclusion because we do not have good tests for this nerve, but we can typically rule out other nerve problems. One way this can be distinguished from other problems is to carefully check the sensation of the front of the thigh. If the medial thigh is numb as well as the lateral thigh, the patient is more likely to have radiculopathy or femoral neuropathy. If the patient has weakness, this is unlikely meralgia paresthetica as the nerve has no motor innervation.

As a purely sensory nerve, the lateral femoral cutaneous nerve is small and easily irritated. This irritation often occurs in patients with elastic compression in their underwear that presses on the area, an object in the pocket of tight pants, or a large belly that hangs down and compresses the nerve. Lateral femoral cutaneous neuropathy used to be called strawberry picker's palsy because one has to crouch down and bend at the hip to pick berries. This motion compresses the nerve at the groin. Treatment involves removing or avoiding the offending agent and stretching the anterior thigh muscles.

Femoral neuropathy results in numbness of the front of the leg below the knee and weakness of the muscles that bend the hip and straighten the knee. This large nerve travels with the femoral artery and vein. Due to this location, it can be injured with vascular procedures. A common procedure for patients who have chest pain is catheterization to access the coronary arteries. During this procedure, a tiny plastic tube is inserted into the femoral artery or vein to thread instrumentation that will give information about the coronary arteries. Just like the blood supply of an injured bone or muscle is important to help with injury healing, the blood supply around the heart is important to feed the pump function of the heart. If one of the three main coronary arteries becomes blocked, this could cause a heart attack or myocardial infarction. *Myocardial infarction* refers to death of the cardiac tissue when the blood supply is cut off. This is similar to avascular necrosis, in which the bone cells die due to inadequate blood supply. Obviously, complications from myocardial infarction are far more dangerous.

Bleeding in the local area of the femoral blood vessels after a catheterization procedure can cause compression of the femoral nerve. For this reason, a pressure dressing is applied and patients are carefully monitored in the hospital after catheterization. Bleeding from inside the abdomen can collect in an open space called the retroperineum. Since the nerve passes through this space, it can get compressed there as well. In regard to sports injuries, this nerve could be injured with a direct blow to the groin in contact sports. Although not common, this is an important diagnosis to consider in patients with hip weakness and nerve pain.

KNEE

As the lower limb corollary to the elbow, the knee also functions as a hinge joint. The bones of the knee are the femur, the tibia, and the fibula. The femur is the longest bone in the body. It articulates with the hip joint as previously mentioned. The tibia is the large bone that makes up the shin. The fibula is a smaller bone on the outside of the tibia that runs from the outside of the knee to the outside of the ankle joint. In physics, long lever arms allow for greater force generation. Since the knee is between the two long bones of the femur and the tibia, the knee is subject to greater forces and subsequent greater injury potential.

Although the size of these bones allows for large forces about the soft tissues of the knee, it does offer some relative protection from fracture. In most athletes, a significant force is required to fracture the bones of the knee. Ligamentous and meniscal injuries are much more common than fractures in this population. If the tibia or femur does break, tear of the cruciate ligaments often accompanies this injury. Fractures of the fibula may be associated with hamstring injury.

The largest of the hamstring muscles, called the biceps femoris, attaches to the head of the fibula. This muscle functions to bend the knee just as the large biceps of the upper limb bends the elbow. A significant blow to this muscle could cause an acute avulsion fracture of the fibular head. When a chip of bone is pulled off a by its attachment to muscle, this is called an avulsion fracture. Since the knee cannot be casted, treatment usually involves splinting, protected weight-bearing, and physical therapy. Surgery is indicated if the fracture is out of place or puts pressure on the blood vessels or nerves.

Avulsion fractures can be both acute and chronic. Osgood Schlatter disease is a condition that occurs in athletes ages eleven to fourteen that represents a chronic avulsion fracture of the tibial tubercle. The tibial tubercle is the bony prominence in the front of the tibia just below the knee joint. It can be palpated in normal patients. In patients with Osgood Schlatter, it appears tender, swollen, and may become very large. This condition presents more frequently in young boys. It is thought to be the result of tiny chronic avulsion fractures from the patellar tendon pulling on this tubercle. This is very a sensitive area in preteens because it contains a center of ossification or growth plate. Treatment involves avoidance of strenuous sports activity, especially activity involving deep knee bends. Fortunately, this heals on its own with activity restriction. Typically, young athletes grow out of this condition.

The knee is also remarkable in regard to the inclusion of a sesamoid bone as part of the joint. The term sesamoid comes from the Greek word for a grain of sesame. These typically tiny bones have the shape of a seed. They occur in the hands and feet and remain of little consequence unless they become inflamed in a condition aptly called sesamoiditis. They function to help the tendons glide more smoothly. The largest sesamoid bone in the body is the patella. It remains as a large seed-shaped bone in front of the femur and tibia.

The muscles in the front of the thigh can generate even more force because of the patella. The quadriceps muscles use the patella as a pulley to function more efficiently. The patella is embedded inside the large conjoined tendon of this group of muscles containing the rectus femoris, vastus medialis, vastus intermedius, and vastus lateralis. The patella improves knee function in two ways: enhancing strength and decreasing injury. By increasing the length of the quadriceps muscles, this increases their ability to generate a force. Stronger quadriceps muscles straighten the knee even better. Tendons that lie up against a hard surface, such as bone, are subject to shearing stresses from that hard surface. The patella lifts the quadriceps tendon so it does not lie directly against the femur when the knee is bent. This decreases the force at an area that is vulnerable to injury. This group of large muscles together with the thick patellar tendon and the patella itself is called the extensor mechanism of the knee after its function.

The extensor mechanism of the knee is susceptible to both acute and chronic sports injury. Acute injury occurs when the patella dislocates. The majority of patellar dislocations occur laterally or away from the midline of the lower limbs. This type of dislocation is clearly visible on inspection. The kneecap is on the side of the leg instead of in the front of the knee. This causes significant pain and swelling.

To treat the dislocation, the patella must be put back into place. Straightening the leg and pushing the patella back toward the center will achieve reduction. An immobilizer may be helpful to keep swelling down and provide stability. Radiographs are necessary to make sure there were no associated fractures. If there is no fracture, early range of motion is recommended to prevent stiffness. Patients with a congenital predisposition to dislocate may be treated operatively and then with quadriceps strengthening. Patients with normal anatomy are usually treated with quadriceps strengthening only.

Chronic dysfunction of the extensor mechanism is far more common. The factors affecting patellar tracking include the shape of the patella itself, the depth of the groove that it sits in, the elasticity of the soft tissues, and the strength of the quadriceps muscles. In recurrent patellar dislocation, it is important to address the whole patient. Patients who have wider hips have a tendency toward the knock-knee position. This inward angle of the knee predisposes the patella to slip out laterally. Because we cannot change the patella itself or the shape of the socket that it sits in, rehabilitation focuses on strengthening the quadriceps muscles and the hip abductors. These muscles tend to be weaker in women, presumably due to their wider hips.

If the kneecap slips out more than the patient can tolerate or if subsequent joint damage has occurred from the dislocation, surgical options should be discussed. These include joint modifications to realign the extensor mechanism of the knee. Care must be taken in children as the tibial tubercle is an open growth plate and the conjoined tendon of this extensor mechanism inserts here. Manipulation of the growth plate can lead to poor outcomes. Surgical treatment typically involves a lateral release. This procedure involves cutting the tight lateral retinaculum that is thought to be pulling the kneecap to the outside. Other surgical treatments are individualized to the patient. Post-operative rehabilitation takes months and involves quadriceps strengthening.

Sometimes, the knee cap tracks poorly without truly dislocating. The best case scenario is when this occurs without any associated patellar dislocation or damage to the knee joint. We refer to this as patellofemoral pain syndrome. Patients typically complain of pain in the front of the knee under the knee cap. Theatre sign is when the patient has worse pain after sitting for long periods of time as if watching a movie. The only finding on physical exam is a "J" sign or slight maltracking of the patella toward the end of knee range of motion when straightening the knee. Patellofemoral pain syndrome can be especially frustrating for patients as imaging is often negative.

Although patients may be relieved to hear their imaging is negative, they often become annoyed to learn there is no easy fix to this persistent problem. The best treatment is aggressive quadriceps strengthening. Sometimes, taping or bracing is used to improve patellar tracking. The taping method used is called McConnell taping and functions to prevent lateral tilt of the knee cap. Braces attempt to provide a bumper against the patella to prevent it from going too far sideways. Although neither method corrects the underlying biomechanics, both can be helpful for symptomatic relief of pain during sports activities.

Another potential sports injury that involves the extensor mechanism of the knee is quadriceps or patellar tendon rupture. When this injury occurs above the knee cap, it is called quadriceps rupture. When the same condition occurs below the knee cap, the term used is patellar tendon rupture. Both injuries refer to a break in the continuity of the extensor mechanism. This may happen as a result of a forceful contraction of the quadriceps to break the impact of the fall. Swelling and bruising is usually apparent. The patient may describe a feeling of instability and may not be able to extend the knee. This usually occurs in athletes between the ages of thirty and sixty. Diagnosis is typically made by MRI. Treatment involves surgical repair of the tendon or muscle.

Just as rupture can occur above or below the patella, tendinopathy can occur in these locations as well. This particular sports injury is called jumper's knee as it is more common in athletes who perform jumping sports, such as basketball, tennis, track, and volleyball. It can happen in older athletes if they have not been training for awhile, and then they run a race or play a game of basketball. Tenderness is apparent on exam. Pain worsens with knee extension under resistance. Treatment involves relative rest from the offending activity. Unlike other some other musculoskeletal conditions, steroids should be avoided in jumper's knee as this can lead to quadriceps tendon rupture. A strap worn around the knee below the patella can be helpful for symptomatic treatment of patellar tendinopathy.

The menisci are two semi-circular pieces of fibrocartilage located in between the thigh bone and the shin bone. The rounded prominences that make up the part of the femur that articulates with the tibia are the condyles. Since the tibia is pretty flat at the top, the menisci fill in the void between the two bones. Looking downward on the knee, the medial meniscus appears in the shape of the letter "C." It is tethered to the MCL and the joint capsule. The lateral meniscus sits just next to the medial meniscus in the shape of an "O." The lateral meniscus attaches to the tendon of the popliteus muscle, making it more mobile than the medial meniscus. The outer portion of the meniscus enjoys an adequate blood supply. The inner two-thirds do not possess an acceptable blood supply. For this reason, the inner portion of the meniscus typically does not heal well and cannot be surgically repaired.

Athletes with meniscal tear will usually recall a trauma prior to the onset of pain. Sometimes, there is an audible "pop" sound during the injury. The mechanism of injury often involves a twisting or over-bending of the knee. Since the mechanism of injury is similar to that of an anterior cruciate ligament injury, meniscal tears occur with ACL tears one-third of the time in young athletes. They are more common in men in their twenties. Patients typically complain of pain along the joint line and may have clicking or locking if there is a loose fragment. The joint line is an imaginary line drawn below the patella but above the tibia. Physical exam tests exist but are limited in specificity. The *McMurray test* involves bending the knee and either internally or externally rotating the shin while simultaneously extending the knee. External rotation challenges the medial meniscus and internal rotation challenges the lateral meniscus. The test is considered positive if there is pain in the area of the meniscus or a palpable "clunk." MRI is typically obtained for accurate diagnosis.

Treatment of meniscal tear depends on the location, severity, and age of the patient. Tears on the outside of the meniscus will likely heal given their adequate blood supply. These patients can be treated with anti-inflammatories, physical therapy, and activity restriction. Running, cutting, and jumping should be avoided for at least eight weeks. Tears toward the inside may need to be surgically repaired, especially if they are accompanied by mechanical symptoms. These symptoms interfere with joint motion. With meniscal tears, this typically refers to clicking or locking. Repairs can be made arthroscopically. The piece that is loose may be removed if it cannot be repaired.

Removal of the meniscus, termed meniscectomy, is controversial in older athletes. Patients in their forties and older may be subject to degenerative tears. These occur with no inciting trauma, but may carry the same symptoms as the acute tears. The reason for the controversy is that removal of the meniscus leads to increased forces on the joint surface. These increased forces in turn lead to knee osteoarthritis. Surgical options are discussed with the patient and decision to treat depends on the functional status of the patient. In older athletes without inciting trauma, physical therapy should always be the initial treatment unless the patient is unable to straighten the knee.

Injury to the anterior cruciate ligament of the knee remains infamous as a catastrophic sports injury. The New England Patriots quarterback, Tom Brady, reportedly tore this ligament at the beginning of the 2008 football season after direct contact to his knee. He was struck at the knee by the shoulder of an opposing player and suffered tears of both the ACL and the MCL. He did not play for the entire subsequent season. Of the four knee ligaments, the ACL is the most commonly injured. The mechanism of injury for contact ACL injuries is usually a blow to the side of the knee with a significant force when the knee is planted.

Noncontact ACL injuries may also occur. This means that the knee was injured by a particular movement as opposed to a blow to the knee. These are more common in female athletes. The mechanism involves an abrupt change in direction when the knee is planted as if in quick pivot away from an opponent. Rapid acceleration or deceleration when running can also tax the ACL. Sports that involve this type of cutting and running motion are soccer, football, and skiing. As such, these are the sports during which we see the most ACL tears.

Multiple theories exist regarding the higher incidence of ACL tears in women. Women are generally more flexible than men due to hormonal changes that occur in puberty. This is thought to be evolutionary so that women can have the experience of the stretching of their pelvic structures to accommodate a baby. We do know that hormone-mediated changes occur during childbirth causing laxity of the ligaments. Noncontact ACL tears are thought to occur in women more frequently related to this propensity for laxity, which has no corollary in men.

Remarkably, women do not have increased ACL tears at a point in their menstrual cycle when their female hormone levels are elevated. The level of hormones in the blood does not seem to correlate with the tendency to tear. When we give women exogenous hormones, as in oral contraceptives, this does not afford protection from ACL injuries. As such, it makes it difficult to conclude that this problem is solely related to hormones. Other theories for the tendency to tear include the shape of the femoral notch and neuromuscular imbalances. The femoral notch has the appearance of a key hole and allows the passage of the ACL. If the walls of the keyhole are too jagged or the hole itself is too small, this is thought to lead to ACL tear. Female patients with ACL tear may exhibit a more sharply cut femoral notch, but the mechanism of injury is not usually from shearing at the notch. Consequently, there are arguments both for and against this notch theory.

The final theory of neuromuscular imbalance in women seems the most plausible and is fortunately a modifiable risk factor. Women have weaker medial quadriceps muscles and weaker hamstrings. In general, women are not as strong as men after changes occur in puberty that redistribute body fat and prepare women for pregnancy. These changes do not tell the whole story. Women have wider hips than men. The knees have a greater tendency to point inward in women than men. This combination puts the quadriceps muscles at a mechanical disadvantage. In particular, the vastus medialis (medial quadriceps muscle) is shortened at this angle and cannot function as efficiently. Also, women have a higher quadriceps to hamstring ratio than men for reasons we do not completely understand.

Given what we know about these neuromuscular imbalances in female athletes, this theory was put to the test with an injury prevention program. Over 1,400 athletes participated in this study. The injury prevention program was developed with women in mind and included exercises that would strengthen the quadriceps and hamstring muscles. These activities included lunges, jumping and landing with the knees pointing forward, and running activities. The overall incidence of ACL injuries was 1.7 times less. The most remarkable difference was seen with noncontact ACL injuries. These became 3.3 times less in the athletes who underwent the aggressive injury prevention program.

The ACL forms a cross with the posterior cruciate ligament (PCL). It starts on the outer portion of the femur and crosses over to end on the inner portion of the tibia. Its function is to keep the shin bone from sliding too far forward. Conversely, it prevents the thigh bone from sliding too far backward and the knee joint from bending backward. The ligament is stretched when the knee is straightened and becomes loose when the knee is bent. If the ACL is torn, the patient tends to over-straighten (or hyperextend) the knee when walking. This action puts more stress on the back portion of the menisci.

On physical exam, patients with ACL tears tend to have significant swelling. This is typically not a subtle injury. Many patients with ACL tears cannot straighten their knees due to the large amount of swelling. It is extremely difficult to examine the ligaments acutely when pain and swelling are present. Regardless, physical exam maneuvers exist to assess the ACL. The Lachman test is performed with the patient lying face up on the exam table. The examiner bends the knee and tries to pull the tibia forward while pushing the femur backward. The test is positive if the tibia can be pulled forward on the affected limb. It is imperative to check the unaffected knee as women tend to have more laxity than men and most patients have some degree of laxity at baseline.

The anterior drawer test is easier to perform than Lachman test, but it may not be as helpful. A negative test may occur even when there is an ACL tear. This test is performed with the knee bent and the foot against the exam table. This position gives the hamstrings a chance to fire and prevent the tibia from moving forward. A positive test occurs if the examiner is able to pull the tibia forward on the affected side more so than on the unaffected side.

Treatment of ACL tear depends on the degree of the tear and the activity level of the patient. If the ligament is completely torn, surgery is usually necessary. If it is stretched without a complete tear, pain control and a good rehabilitation program may be all that is necessary. Pain control is typically with anti-inflammatories to help reduce the associated swelling. Also, compression splints and ice can be helpful for swelling. Narcotic medications may be given for severe pain. Since both the ACL and the hamstrings restrict anterior or forward motion of the tibia, exercise management of ACL injury focuses on hamstring strengthening. Once that is achieved, the athlete can progress to proprioceptive exercises that challenge the stability of the joint.

The ACL and PCL form a cross that can be seen when looking inside the knee with the patient facing forward. For this reason, the term cruciate is used to describe these ligaments. As such, the PCL must run from the medial femur to the lateral tibia. Unlike ACL injuries, PCL injuries rarely occur without contact. The PCL is the strongest of the four knee ligaments. Since it takes so much to tear this ligament, the injury may be missed initially while the physician is caring for other life-threatening injuries. Patients with PCL tears typically have been through polytrauma, such as a car accident. They may have swelling of the brain, lung puncture, or abdominal bleeding. Doctors are focusing so heavily on keeping the patient alive, the PCL injury may not be diagnosed right away. Once this injury is discovered, surgical consult is obtained, as there is still disagreement as to how to treat PCL injuries.

Diagnosis of a PCL tear can be made on physical exam once swelling has subsided. Since this ligament keeps the tibia from sliding backward, this action occurs in the absence of the ligament. This becomes obvious on clinical exam with the thumb sign. In a normal knee, the examiner can fit one thumb on top of the tibia on either side of the patella, as if it were a small shelf. When this shelf is absent, this is the sign that the tibia has sunk backward and the PCL is torn.

Usually, PCL injuries are managed similarly to ACL injuries with one exception, they progress to surgery less frequently. It is possible, although not desirable, to participate in athletics with a chronic tear of the PCL. Initially, recommendations include protected weight-bearing, rest, ice, compression, and elevation. Early range of motion is encouraged to prevent stiffness. Physical therapy involves strengthening the quadriceps and hamstring muscles. The controversy is regarding both when to operate and what operation to perform. The best approach is one that is individualized to the specific patient and the skill level of the surgeon. Most surgeons will agree that if there is an associated ligamentous tear or fracture, surgery may be necessary. The controversy exists because patients can function without a PCL. We know this from a study done in the early days of MRI.

One year, all the players at the NFL pre-draft physicals were given an MRI of their knee as part of this study. These are some of our nation's most talented athletes who run and jump regularly. Surprisingly, there was a 2 percent incidence of PCL tears. These were isolated PCL tears in athletes with no knee pain or problems. Given the high functional level of these individuals, it is difficult to know when surgery is the best option. As such, surgery is reserved for patients with persistent and debilitating symptoms or other injuries that clearly necessitate intervention.

Injuries to the MCL and the LCL do not get the media attention of the infamous ACL since they may occur with other problems that are more serious. When they do occur in isolation, there may be little swelling and they may not need surgical treatment. The MCL runs from the medial femoral condyle to the inside of the tibia. Injury may occur with a blow to the outside of the bent knee, as this puts too much stress on the inside part of the knee. The LCL runs from the lateral femoral condyle and attaches to the outside of the fibula. Injury may occur with a blow to the inside of the bent knee. This type of contact puts too much tension on the soft tissues at the outside of the knee when the knee is planted against the ground.

These ligamentous injuries are treated in the context of other injuries sustained. O'Donoghue's unhappy triad refers to injury of the MCL, ACL, and medial meniscus when seen together. We used to think that the MCL was more commonly injured with the ACL and the medial meniscus. Now, we know that the LCL or lateral meniscus may be injured concurrently just as frequently depending on the location of the forces at the time of injury. Regardless, these injuries are treated with rest, ice, compression, and elevation with early range of motion and gradual return to activity after quadriceps strengthening.

Iliotibial band syndrome is a common knee tendinopathy in runners. As previously mentioned, this band of fascia and muscle runs from the top of the hip to the outside of the tibia and inserts on an outpouching of bone called Gerdy tubercle on the lateral aspect of the tibia. When the knee goes from straight to bent, it slides over the lateral femoral condyle. This condition may be related to overuse during running or from tightness of the muscle itself. Generally, it responds to stretching. To stretch the iliotibial band, the patient can stand with the affected leg crossed in front of the unaffected leg. While holding on to a bar or the wall, the patient should lean their trunk away from the affected limb. They should feel stretch along the outside of the leg. Some runners find benefit with rolling a piece of circular foam or a tennis ball over the muscle to break up fibrosis.

There are multiple bursae about the knee. Clinically important bursae include the prepatellar, suprapatellar, infrapatellar, pes anserine, and posterior bursa. The most commonly damaged bursa is the prepatellar bursa, which lies between the knee cap and the skin. Bursitis at this location may come from crawling on the hands and knees. As such, inflammation at this site is called housemaid's knee. As expected, the suprapatellar bursa and the infrapatellar bursa are above and below the patella respectively. The suprapatellar bursa may communicate with the joint capsule. As such, it may become painful when the joint is inflamed. The mechanism of injury in infrapatellar bursitis typically involves kneeling upright as if in praying. For this reason, this type of bursitis is called vicar's knee. It may be difficult to distinguish these bursitides from knee joint problems. Careful palpation can sometimes sort out the location of pain given the superficial location of the bursae. Bursitis is typically very tender to the touch and may exhibit redness, warmth, or swelling.

The pes anserine bursa is outside and medial to the knee joint. It is named for the sartorius, gracilis, and semitendinosis tendons that insert there. The sartorius is called the *tailor muscle* because it functions in sitting cross-legged as if sewing clothes while sitting on the floor. The gracilis helps to bring the thighs together and bend the knee. The semitendinosis assists in straightening the hip and bending the knee. The tendon of the semitendinosis can be felt on the medial side of the back of the knee when pressing the heel into the floor with the knee bent. These are all fairly thin muscles in comparison to the quadriceps, adductors, and biceps femoris of the thigh. The three tendons are supposed to have the appearance of a goose's foot and are located adjacent to the MCL.

The pes anserine bursa often becomes inflamed in athletes who have tight hamstrings. Often, this can be treated with a hamstring stretching program. The final bursa is the posterior or popliteal bursa, which refers to the back of the knee joint. This bursa communicates with the joint cavity and extends backward between the cavity and the top of the calf muscle called the gastrocnemius. This bursa can become very prominent, to the point where a large fluid collection is seen in the back of the knee. This may be from overuse activity or injury to the soft tissue, creating increased fluid that tracks backward. The appearance of this fluid-filled cavity is termed a Baker cyst. Unlike the other bursae, a Baker cyst may rupture. Although it is a form of bursitis, it may not be painful at onset like the other bursidities. Rupture of the cyst is not typically dangerous, but it provokes extreme pain in the back of the knee. Once the ruptured fluid has resorbed over hours and days, the pain diminishes. Baker cysts can be aspirated, but the pocket of fluid usually returns due to the continued presence of the underlying lining that was created by the cyst or increased synovial fluid from associated arthritis or soft tissue injury.

Most bursitis is treated topically. Ice can be exceptionally helpful. Sometimes, iontophoresis can be helpful for inflammation. Iontophoresis is the process involving a physical therapist applying corticosteroids to the skin and using an electric pad that sends tiny waves of electricity to pulse the steroid into the area of inflammation. This is usually well tolerated as it does not involve any injections and rarely leads to side effects. Since the bursa is just under skin, it tends to work well for pain. In some patients with dark skin tones, there may be a slight decrease in skin pigment in the area of the steroid application. Some patients do not like the sensation of the tiny electric waves, but most patients feel that it helps with pain. Injury of the skin does not typically occur with this low level of electricity.

Osteoarthritis of the knee is a common cause of disability in the United States. Patients typically complain of pain with weight-bearing and stiffness on awakening or after sitting. They may have knee swelling. Eventually, the pain may progress to the point that it is difficult to bend or straighten the knee. Due to the unique aspect of the patella as part of the joint, the knee is divided into three compartments. Arthritis is described in terms of the compartment that it occupies.

Since osteoarthritis is degenerative, the wearing away of cartilage tends to occur in areas where the bone is closest together. This makes it easier for the surfaces to rub against each other. Since the tibiofemoral joint is the one that absorbs the weight during walking, this joint is commonly affected by osteoarthritis. The medial and lateral compartments refer to the inside and outside parts of this joint, or where the tibia articulates with the femur in standing. Medial compartment arthritis occurs more in patients who have knees that are bow-legged, and lateral compartment arthritis occurs more in patients who have knees that bend inward. The wearing away tends to occur on the inside of the angle formed by the knee malalignment. In patients who are bow-legged or have varus alignment, more force is put on the medial compartment. The opposite is true in patients with valgus alignment or knock-knee deformity.

The patellofemoral joint is where the patella meets the femur. Arthritis at this joint may occur from improper tracking of the patella. The cartilage on the back of the patella begins to wear away in a condition termed chondromalacia patellae. Typically, the patella tracks too far to the outside or lateral aspect of the knee. For this reason, therapy is focused on strengthening the medial quadriceps muscle, termed the vastus medialis, to pull the knee back the other way. If the condition progresses, it may lead to patellofemoral compartment osteoarthritis. Surgical treatment depends on the extent of the arthritis.

Arthritis can be diagnosed easily with radiographs. However, standing views are necessary to exclude early arthritis. The reason for this is that arthritis is usually judged by joint space narrowing. This is first apparent when bearing weight. Most radiographs are performed with the patient lying down. Early narrowing of the joint space cannot be seen on these views. Other clues to osteoarthritis on radiographs include sclerosis and subchondral cysts. Sclerosis is a brightness of the bone in the area that the cartilage is worn away. Subchondral cysts are fluid-filled sacs under the first layer of bone that form from the rubbing that occurs after the cartilage is worn away. For patellofemoral compartment osteoarthritis, a special x-ray view is obtained. This is called a sunrise view because the knee cap is visualized on top of the femoral condyles as if it were the sun over a mountain.

Surgical treatment depends on the location of the arthritis. For arthritis in one compartment, a partial knee replacement may be done. This is done if there is marked joint space narrowing on x-ray in one compartment, but the other areas are relatively preserved. Multi-compartment arthritis usually requires a total knee replacement. A total knee replacement involves replacing the surfaces of the femur, tibia, and underside of the knee cap. The replacement parts are usually made of metal, ceramic, or plastic. Typically, the metal used in orthopedic implants is safe to go through an MRI machine. However, it is important to note than even metal that does not interfere with the magnetic properties of the MRI may distort the image.

After knee replacement, rehabilitation is necessary for the best outcome. Initially, this consists of range of motion exercise to mobilize swelling and prevent stiffness and contracture. Later, gentle exercises are performed to strengthen the quadriceps and the hamstrings. Eventually, more aggressive exercises are recommended that mimic the patient's prior activity level. Stair climbing is an important hurdle for most patients. Recommendations for athletic activity depend on the procedure and the surgeon.

Doctors like to base their recommendations on evidence. Since joint replacements have not been around for that long, we do not have great long-term data on activity after joint replacement. Study of athletic activity after joint replacement is largely based on surveys, and recommendations vary depending on the prior activity level of the patient. Prior to the procedure, it is important for the athlete to have a frank discussion with the surgeon about expectations regarding athletic activities after joint replacement. In general, the following sports are permitted after knee replacement: bowling, stationary and road cycling, ballroom dancing, golf, horseback riding, shuffleboard, swimming, canoeing, hiking, and speed walking. Contact sports such as baseball, basketball, football, hockey, soccer, racquetball, and handball are not recommended. Because running and jumping may impact wear or loosening of the prosthesis, some surgeons do not permit jogging, singles tennis, and volleyball. Rock climbing has generally been discouraged, but permission for skiing depends on the type of skiing and the previous experience of the patient.

Although contracture after joint replacement is not unique to the knee, it is important to highlight because of the importance of knee flexion in any athletic activity. Other potential complications are similar to those with hip replacement. Contracture refers to a scarring and fibrosis of the soft tissue that may occur after joint replacement. This can be a particularly difficult problem to treat because it is a fixed deformity; it is not from tight muscles that need to be stretched. Once the scar tissue has formed, stretching may not reverse the process. Since everyday walking requires bending and straightening the knee, contracture will make it difficult for the patient to walk. If the patient cannot walk or climb stairs, athletic activity may not be an option. As such, the possibility of contracture is an important argument for early and aggressive rehabilitation after joint replacement.

The most common entrapment neuropathy of the knee affects the peroneal nerve. The common peroneal nerve is a branch of the sciatic nerve that comes off at the side of the knee. It winds around the head of the fibula. At this point, it is very superficial and can sometimes be palpated when swollen. It is subject to compression as it runs under the peroneus longus muscle, which tethers the nerve to the fibular head. Then, it runs on the outside of the calf muscle to provide sensation to the skin on the outside of the calf. After this, the common peroneal nerve divides into two main branches, the deep peroneal and superficial peroneal nerves.

The deep peroneal nerve innervates the anterior muscles of the leg by traveling under the peroneus longus. This nerve supplies the muscles that control foot dorsiflexion and toe extension. The tibialis anterior is the strongest contributor to foot dorsiflexion. Also, the deep peroneal nerve provides sensation to the area between the big toe and the second toe. The superficial peroneal nerve provides sensation to most of the top of the foot and side of the shin. (Of note, there is a small area of sensation on the outside of the foot that is supplied by the sural nerve.) It also innervates two small muscles on the outside of the calf which help turn the ankle outward, the peroneal longus and brevis.

The superficial location of the peroneal nerve at the level of the head of the fibula renders it particularly vulnerable to trauma at this area. Although fracture of the fibula is more likely to cause problems for this nerve, peroneal neuropathy has been reported with tibial fracture as well. Ligamentous rupture in the knee may cause peroneal nerve injury. The ACL was the most commonly reported ligament rupture with peroneal neuropathy in one series (Krinckas 2000). Remarkably, peroneal neuropathy can also occur with ankle injury. The peroneal muscles keep the ankle from turning inward. In ankle sprain, these muscles get stretched. Since the nerve is tethered by the peroneus longus at the knee, injury to the nerve may occur when the ankle is turned inward and this muscle tightens to absorb the impact.

The other branch off of the sciatic nerve at the knee is the tibial nerve. This nerve passes deep in the back of the knee with the blood vessels to innervate the calf muscles. Then, it passes under a band of fascia called the flexor retinaculum to innervate one ankle muscle and muscles in the foot as well as the skin of the bottom of the foot. Since this nerve is buried deep under the muscles and soft tissue of the back of the knee, it is rarely injured at this location. The tibial nerve at the knee should be evaluated if the athlete receives a sharp blow to the back of the knee, such as an accidental kick in soccer, or if there is vascular injury. Since the nerve runs close to the blood vessels, it should be evaluated for concurrent damage in rare cases of vascular compromise.

Sometimes, pain at the knee does not come from the knee at all. A pinched L3 nerve in the lumbar spine can cause burning and tingling isolated to the front of the knee. If there is a sensory deficit over the anterior knee, this diagnosis is more likely. An inversion ankle injury can cause peroneal neuropathy at the lateral knee or proximal peroneal tendon injury. Painful hip osteoarthritis can cause thigh pain that may radiate to the knee just as painful knee osteoarthritis may radiate to the hip. If the patient's complaints are non-specific, both joints should be examined to increase diagnostic yield.

ANKLE AND FOOT

The bones of the ankle form a tunnel through which the foot bones rest. The tibia forms one side and the roof of the tunnel. The fibula forms the other side of the tunnel. The talus rests in the middle of the tunnel. Together with the tibia and fibula, the talus forms the true ankle joint. The prominence of bone on the medial aspect of the ankle is the medial malleolus of the tibia. The prominence on the outside of the ankle is the lateral malleolus of the fibula. The talus rests on the large bone that comprises the heel, termed the calcaneus, which is the bone that the patient lands on when jumping.

Since we cover our feet with shoes that have a flat bottom, most people perceive that their feet are uniformly in contact with the ground. In fact, the talus and calcaneous form the beginnings of a construct that becomes the arch of the foot. This concept is best illustrated by thinking about bare footsteps in sand. Footprints on the beach are largely comprised of the lateral portion of the foot. This is because the bones of the foot form a three-dimensional arch, and we actually only walk on the outside portion of this arch. The largest bone in the foot is the calcaneus, or heel bone. This bone articulates with the cuboid bone. The talus is above and next to the calcaneus, closer to the inside part of the arch. The talus articulates with the navicular bone. The three wedge-shaped cuneiforms articulate with the navicular and make up the medial portion of the arch. The phalanges are the bones that make up the toes, and the metatarsals are the bones in between. Although all the bones are part of the foot, body weight is distributed only between the calcaneus and metarsals. These bones are the opposite ends of the arch that make contact with the floor.

The unique structure of the ankle and foot would not be possible without the ligaments on either side of the ankle and throughout the foot. The medial or deltoid ligament is on the inside part of the ankle and restricts the inward motion of the ankle, termed inversion, which is the motion that would occur if the patient were trying to look at the bottom of his or her foot. Three ligaments make up the lateral ligament of the ankle, which restricts ankle eversion, which refers to turning the ankle out and up. These three ligaments are the anterior talofibular, the posterior talofibular, and the calcaneofibular ligament. There is another ligament between the two shin bones called the tibiofibular ligament that functions to maintain the integrity of the joint space. Compromise of this ligament could result in widening of the ankle mortise.

Fractures of the foot and ankle can be devastating not only for the limitations in walking, but also for the potential complications that may arise from bearing weight through our arms. Ankle fractures can occur in the tibia or the fibula. Since these two bones form a tunnel for the talus, it becomes a huge problem if there is a fracture in both bones as it disrupts the integrity of the tunnel. This type of fracture is called a bimalleolar or trimalleolar fracture after the malleoli or protuberances of bone on either side of the tunnel that contains the talus. Since both bimalleolar and trimalleolar fractures are unstable, they typically require surgical intervention.

The talus and calcaneus of the hindfoot are relatively resistant to fracture. Severe trauma, such as a motor vehicle collision or a fall from a height can fracture these bones. If a patient lands in a standing position from a significant fall, the calcaneus absorbs much of the force. The talus is a bone with tenuous blood supply. Although uncommon during regular sports activity, fractures of the talus or calcaneus tend to set the patient up for arthritis later in life.

Metatarsal fractures are more common in sports injury. The fifth (outermost) metatarsal may fracture with the inversion injury sustained in ankle sprain. Although most fractures of the metatarsals can be managed nonoperatively, patients with fifth metatarsal fracture should have an orthopedic surgery consult. Fractures in certain parts of this bone have a high rate of poor healing, called nonunion or delayed union. These types of fractures need surgical intervention.

A stress fracture is a type of fracture that occurs without a significant acute trauma. Stress fractures come in two varieties: fatigue fractures and insufficiency fractures. Fatigue fractures happen after a normal bone has been exposed to a repeated stress. The stress builds up over time and eventually the bone gives way to fracture. An example of this type of fracture may occur in a female runner who increases her distance repeatedly and does not take a break between marathons. The bones of the feet and shins are only constructed to take so much pounding. Eventually, a fracture may occur in this otherwise healthy runner without an acute trauma because bone remodeling cannot keep up with bone breakdown.

Insufficiency fractures happen in people with weak bones even without an abnormal force. The most common example of this is a patient with osteoporosis. When the bone is fragile, a fracture can occur even in a fall from standing. Typically, this type of trip and fall would not cause a fracture in a patient with normal bone structure. In osteoporosis, the bone structure is weak and it just takes a little force to induce a fracture. The most common osteoporosis-type fractures occur in the spine and hip, but they can occur in the feet as well. Osteoporosis is rare in athletes as weight-bearing exercise has a protective effect on the bones.

In general, osteoporosis tends to occur in women over age sixty-five because of a decrease in estrogen. Estrogen has a protective effect on the bones. As this female hormone declines, bone health may decline along with it. Other causes of poor bone health include kidney disease, rheumatologic illness, and prior prolonged oral steroid use. Currently, there are many medicines available to combat this decline as discussed in the spine section. Radiographs should always be obtained in patients with bone tenderness and risk factors for osteoporosis.

Remarkably, stress fractures may not show up on initial radiographs. If x-rays are negative and a stress fracture is suspected, a bone scan or an MRI should be obtained. These tests are more sensitive for stress fracture. Once this type of fracture is diagnosed, treatment involves avoiding the offending activity. A cast boot may be helpful to immobilize the affected area. In most cases of musculoskeletal injury, nonsteroidal anti-inflammatories are encouraged. The treatment of stress fracture is an exception to this rule for two reasons. Stress fractures typically occur in athletes who are participating in too much activity. If the pain is treated, they may go back to the offending activity too early. Another reason is that anti-inflammatories have been implicated in delayed healing of fractures. As such, ice and Tylenol are typically recommended for pain control. Stress fractures are far more common in the lower limbs. They may occur in the shins as well as the ankle or foot. The large shin bone, or tibia, is a common site of these fractures despite its sturdy appearance. Patients typically complain of pain in the shins that is worse with activity, especially running. Stress fracture is important to rule out in a patient with presumed shin splints. Shin splints or medial tibial stress syndrome refers to activity-related pain in the shins without an associated stress fracture. Some practitioners believe that shin splints are on a continuum with stress fracture, such that they are a manifestation of an early or pre-stress fracture. Activity modifications are recommended for both patients with stress fracture and with shin splints.

Patients can swim, jog in the water, or cycle while they are healing from stress fracture. Since these fractures are rather common among runners, running must be avoided for at least six to eight weeks. Some areas of bone that are prone to poor healing such as the fifth metatarsal or the navicular bones may take even longer or require special interventions to heal. When the patient is pain-free, they may return to light jogging on a limited basis. Successful return to activity depends on a very gradual increase in this activity. Patients have the best outcome when they increase their mileage by no more than 10 percent per week. Although it may be very time-consuming to achieve their prior mileage goals, this is the safest way to prevent further complications from stress fracture.

Another factor that is important in stress fractures is treatment of calcium or vitamin D deficiency. Calcium and vitamin D are important building blocks of bone. Stress fractures heal best when these substrates are available. Deficiency can come from inadequate intake, poor gastrointestinal absorption, or decreased ability to metabolize these agents. In female runners, inadequate intake tends to be a problem. Sometimes, this is from lack of proper nutrition or too much athletic activity without enough time for snacks. Female athletes in the northern states are at a particular risk, as vitamin D is naturally manufactured by the body as a result of sun exposure. Education regarding available sources of calcium and vitamin D and the proper caloric intake for increased athletic activity can combat this problem.

Prevention of stress fractures involves avoidance of rapid increases in training regimen and increasing nutritional intake along with training level. Lack of arch support has also been implicated in stress fracture. As such, orthotics are recommended for patients with flat feet. Since stress fractures have been found in patients who recently changed their running terrain, patients are encouraged to avoid surfaces without shock absorption. For example, running on the treadmill may be easier on the injured part than running on a track. Running on soft surfaces such as grass or gravel may help with stress fracture. Unfortunately, athletes are also far more likely to suffer ankle sprain on this type of surface.

Ankle sprain is the most common sports medicine diagnosis of the ankle. This typically occurs when the patient turns the ankle inward. This inversion injury is commonly seen in contact sports. Basketball reports the most ankle sprains, likely because it involves both running and jumping. Typically, patients complain of pain and swelling on the outside part of the ankle after twisting the ankle inward. For this reason, sprains nearly always occur on the outside of the ankle. Patients do not typically twist the ankle outward. This would be an awkward motion when standing on the toes. As such, the medial ankle ligaments are rarely sprained. The most commonly sprained ligament is the anterior talofibular ligament on the lateral aspect of the ankle.

Once the swelling has developed, it becomes much more difficult to examine the ankle for sprain injury. Often, the examiner will defer these ligamentous tests until the swelling subsides, usually about seven to ten days post-injury. In the anterior drawer test, the examiner pulls the heel anteriorly while grasping the proximal lower limb. In the talar tilt test, the examiner inverts the heel while grasping the proximal limb. These motions are performed in the normal ankle for comparison. If the ligaments stretch more in the injured ankle, the patient is diagnosed with an ankle sprain.

Sprains are graded from one to three. Grade one ankle sprain refers to mild stretching of the ligaments. Grade two ankle sprain indicates moderate stretching of the ligaments. In grade three ankle sprain, the ligament is completely torn off. If the ligament completely gives way on exam, then the patient has a grade three sprain. Casting or surgery may be necessary for these sprains. Only an experienced practitioner can determine between grades one and two with physical exam tests. For mild and moderate sprain, the patient is often treated with splinting.

An air splint with medial and lateral stays that conforms to the patient's ankle is usually prescribed. Since the sprain may not be the only injury present, radiographs are often performed to assess for fracture. Fractures that may occur with the common mechanism of injury in ankle sprain are fifth metatarsal fractures and distal fibular fractures. Although sprains can be even more painful than fractures, it is generally acceptable to put weight on a sprain as tolerated. It is best not to bear weight on a fracture until it has been evaluated and casted or splinted appropriately.

Treatment of ankle sprain includes protected weight-bearing, rest, ice, compression, and elevation. Early mobilization is pivotal to maintain ankle range of motion. If the ankle heals with the ligaments in the stretched-out position (i.e., too much inversion), it can encumber the athlete's return to running. It is recommended to strengthen the muscles on the outside of the calf, called the peroneal muscles, to protect the injured area, and improve running mechanics. As the ankle gets stronger, more challenging therapeutic activities can be prescribed. Proprioceptive training encompasses standing on a balance board or bosu ball and trying to balance. By creating controlled situations where the ankle is put off balance, the athlete can practice dynamic techniques to strengthen the injured area and prevent future ankle sprain.

The reason for the success of this treatment is based on changes that occur at the minute histologic level. Hemorrhage and inflammation begin immediately after injury. In this phase, ice and protected weight-bearing allow time for the body to clear this up. Then, fibroblastic proliferation occurs around two to three days post-injury. Collagen protein formation and subsequent maturation happens over the following weeks. Since collagen is a building block for the ligaments, this helps to heal the injured area. The whole process takes eight to twelve weeks. Some athletes experience instability even months out from the ankle sprain. This is best treated with muscle strengthening.

Strengthening of the peroneal muscles, which serve to evert the ankle, is the best way to prevent this injury. Taping the ankle and ankle braces also prevent recurrent ankle sprain. Taping works better than bracing to control forces, but it breaks down after ten minutes of exercise. A brace provides consistent support throughout athletic activity. Utilization of taping or bracing depends largely on athlete preferences and available resources. The most important concept is to prevent the ankle from turning inward while running or jumping by having strong ankle evertors or physically preventing inversion with an outside mechanical force.

Women are 25 percent more likely to suffer mild (grade one) ankle sprains. We do not know why this is the case, but many specialists theorize that it may have to do with increased ligamentous laxity in women. There is no increased risk in women for ankle sprains of grades two and three. Another theory is that this occurs in women as a result of high heels. These shoes put the ankle in a position of plantar flexion, where it is susceptible to twisting inward. However, this theory is unlikely to be correct because studies have shown that these injuries occur while women are wearing sneakers.

Sensation is important to examine as there could be an associated peroneal neuropathy that occurred during the ankle inversion injury. Both ankle sprain and peroneal neuropathy may lead to weakness of the peroneal musculature. Sensory deficit of the deep peroneal nerve may occur between the great toe and second toe. The superficial peroneal nerve innervates the anterolateral shin. Local lateral malleolar pain is common with ankle sprain. Burning or radiating pain may suggest associated nerve injury.

Turf toe refers to a sprain of the ligaments of the big toe. This can occur if the toe is bent backward or gets driven into the front of the shoe by impact. Turf toe is common in football and soccer players. The term comes from the dilemma of artificial turf. This surface is associated with more injuries that grass, but it is so much easier to maintain. These injuries are graded one to three like ankle sprains. A grade three injury is complete disruption of the ligamentous complex. Swelling and ecchymosis is often present on exam.

Radiographs may be helpful when marked bruising or deformity is present to rule out associated fractures. Treatment involves relative rest of the joint.

Since the big toe needs to bend for normal walking, immobilization in a shoe with a stiff sole may afford some protection to this area. Taping the great toe to the second toe can also provide some support. Serious injuries may require a period of protected weight-bearing with crutch ambulation. These injuries rarely require surgery and often heal in six weeks.

The Achilles tendon is so aptly named for being a weak point in the body. Achilles, a character in Greek mythology, was a very strong war hero. The only weak part of his body was said to be his heel. As it turns out, we all may be a little weak at the heels. This tendon is the conjoined tendon formed by the gastrocnemius and soleus muscles of the calf. These muscles are attached to the calcaneus and function to plantar flex the ankle. Plantar flexion is the ankle motion that occurs when the patient stands on his toes. This is a key action in jumping and cutting sports. As such, patients tend to suffer from Achilles tendon injury after participating in basketball, tennis, or squash.

The Achilles tendon can tear leaving a ball of muscle at the back of the calf. This acute injury is very painful and occurs with landing from a jump or colliding with another player. Commonly, it is described as a feeling of being smacked in the calf with a club. The pain tends to dissipate, but muscle weakness remains. On physical exam, the patient may not be able to stand on her toes. The Thompson test assesses the integrity of the calf muscle-tendon unit. The test involves squeezing the patient's calf and watching for ankle disrupted from a tear in the tendon.

Prompt treatment of Achilles tendon rupture is pivotal in the outcome for the patient. When the tendon tears, the muscle tends to pull toward the back of the knee because it is still attached there. When the muscle starts to heal in this retracted position, it is much more difficult to stretch it back to its original position during surgical repair. If the original position cannot be achieved, the repair may not be possible or the patient may suffer from a subsequent decrease in ankle range of motion. Achilles tendon tear can be treated with surgical repair or immobilization in a cast or brace. As with most tendon tears, treatment depends on the degree of the tear and the activity level of the patient.

Most of the tendons in the body are vulnerable to injury at the area close to their attachment to bone. This area of inflammation is so common, it even has its own name. Enthesitis refers to inflammation of the tendon at its insertion site on bone. The Achilles tendon is unique in that it usually becomes inflamed at an area closer to the muscle belly. Typically, Achilles tendonitis occurs two to six centimeters away from the area where the tendon inserts on the calcaneus.

Pain from Achilles tendinitis occurs in the back of the calf and heel. Although the pain is similar to tendon tear, these are usually easy to distinguish on clinical exam as there is no abnormal continuity of the muscle if it is not torn. There may be swelling or warmth, but there will be no palpable muscle bulge in the back of the calf. Treatment depends on the degree of the disability. If the patient is in a lot of pain, a cast boot may be helpful to encourage the patient to limit activity. Ice and anti-inflammatories may also help. Stretching of the calf muscle is necessary to allow gradual return to activities. A padded heel cup may also provide symptomatic relief. Cortisone injections are not performed as there is evidence of increased Achilles tendon rupture with this procedure.

The posterior tibial tendon wraps around the medial malleolus of the tibia. This muscle functions to invert the ankle. The muscle belly is located deep in the calf, almost in back of the tibia. This tendon is particularly important in that it maintains the integrity of the arch of the foot. On physical exam, patients with a tear of the posterior tibial tendon exhibit the too many toes sign. Acute rupture of this tendon is exceedingly rare. Typically, laxity results in gradual collapse of the arch of the foot. Collapsed arches are more prevalent in athletes over age sixty. Initially, arch supports are helpful for this condition.

Tendinopathy of the tibialis posterior is a more common problem in younger athletes. This results in pain just below the medial malleolus that worsens with resisted ankle inversion. Immobilization in a walking cast boot for ten to fourteen days may be helpful to provide relative rest for the tendon. Stretching can be performed during this period and should be continued throughout the following months. Strengthening should be performed when the pain decreases. Focused ankle strengthening exercise may be helpful to protect this area from activities that require shock absorption. Athletes who do a lot of running often benefit from shoes with an arch support to prevent stress on this tendon.

The peroneal muscles function in ankle eversion. The tendons of the peroneus longus and brevis may be injured in ankle sprain as inversion injury stresses this area. Often, the pain from muscle or tendon injury is secondary to the pain from the ankle sprain itself. Pain from peroneal tendinopathy is also located in the lateral ankle. As such, muscle or tendon injury may not be diagnosed until well after the injury. Fortunately, treatment is similar to the treatment for ankle sprain. A period of immobilization followed by gradual return to activity yields the best results. The athlete should not return to sports activity until he or she is pain-free.

Pain in the heel that occurs first thing in the morning is classic for plantar fasciitis. The plantar fascia is a thick band of connective tissue that fans out from the heel bone to cover the bottom of the foot. The reason the pain occurs with the first steps of the morning has to do with the way we sleep. In resting, our toes flop forward and the ankle relaxes in a plantar flexed position all night long. In the morning, the ankle must dorsiflex (as if bringing the toes back toward the head) to allow for normal ambulation. This position puts tension on the plantar fascia that had been resting in the loose position during the night. In normal patients, this does not typically provoke pain. However, in patients with plantar fasciitis, this increased tension can be excruciating.

Plantar fasciitis can be diagnosed with palpation of the bottom of the foot. If the patient has pain over the calcaneus that was atraumatic in onset and worsens with passive dorsiflexion, then plantar fasciitis is likely. Radiographs may be obtained to rule out calcaneal fracture or other bone problems. Bone spurs at the area where the calcaneus attaches to the plantar fascia are very common. We used to think that these spurs, called osteophytes, were the cause of the patient's foot pain. Now, we think they might be the effect. An inflamed fascial band demonstrates a thickening and contracture. This relative shortening of the plantar fascia results in an increased force at the area where it attaches to bone. This increased force pulls on the bone and causes the spur. Resection of these spurs does not result in decreased pain for the patient.

Plantar fasciitis is increasingly common in runners with flat feet. Treatment involves padding the area with a gel heel cup or insertion of arch supports in patients with flat feet. Stretching of the plantar fascia is necessary in treatment of this condition. Since pain in the morning is very common, night splints have been developed to position the ankle in dorsiflexion during sleep. These splints have the appearance of a ski boot with a kickstand. Although increasingly uncomfortable, especially for the person in bed with the patient, they can be helpful in patients who have trouble stretching on their own. Since the Achilles tendon also attaches to the calcaneus, Achilles tendinopathy can be seen with plantar fasciitis and vice versa. Treatment involves pain control and consistent stretching of the bottom of the foot and calf muscles.

Numbness and tingling of the bottom of the foot her usually attributed to tibial neuropathy. The tibial nerve branches off the sciatic nerve at the back of the knee and remains well protected by soft tissue as it courses down the back of the lower leg. At the ankle, it passes under a band of fascia called the flexor retinaculum to innervate the bottom of the foot. The branches of the tibial nerve that lend sensation to the bottom of the foot are called the medial and lateral plantar nerves for the parts of the bottom of the foot that they cover. Patients with tarsal syndrome complain of numbness and tingling of the bottom of the foot.

Tarsal tunnel syndrome is the name given to compression of the tibial nerve at the flexor retinaculum, just like carpal tunnel refers to compression of the median nerve at the wrist. Unlike carpal tunnel syndrome, tarsal tunnel syndrome is believed by some physicians to be exceedingly rare. The reasons for this may be related to our limited ability to test for tarsal tunnel syndrome and the lack of potential functional compression at this area. Typically, we use electrodiagnostic studies to evaluate for nerve injury. There are several easy ways to evaluate the carpal tunnel with this type of test. Our nerve tests for the tarsal tunnel are simply not as accurate due to anatomical considerations and equipment limitations.

Another important functional consideration in tarsal tunnel syndrome is lack of torque on this nerve. Tension on an irritated nerve will result in worsening of pain. This can be demonstrated in a patient with a pinched nerve of the back by lifting the symptomatic leg toward the ceiling. There may be subtle pressure on this nerve when turning the ankle inward, but nothing like the motion that occurs at the wrist during everyday tasks. For example, it is very easy to look at the palm of your hand. It becomes much more difficult to look at the bottom of the foot. Since there are few activities which challenge the tarsal tunnel, there is likely to be less irritation of this nerve.

HEAD INJURIES

Like spinal cord injury, traumatic brain injury can be devastating to an athlete. These types of injuries occur in contact sports from collisions with another player or with the ball. Football is the most commonly reported sport in athletes who suffer sports-related concussion. Head injuries also occur in skiing, hockey, soccer, and basketball. A concussion is equivalent to a mild traumatic brain injury. The brain is well protected by the skull, but hitting the head can result in neurologic symptoms. Headache is a common obvious complaint. Patients who have sustained a concussion may also experience confusion, dizziness, or trouble with vision, speech, or mood. These symptoms usually get better within seven to ten days. There is great debate about when an athlete can return to play after concussion. The reason for this debate is the catastrophic nature of second impact syndrome.

Remarkably, patients who suffer serious symptoms after a concussion are unlikely to be experiencing their first incident. Second impact syndrome refers to severe neurologic symptoms resulting in disability and even death after a concussion. It is thought to be related to a threshold that is crossed after multiple concussive incidents. Although relatively rare, this syndrome is incredibly scary. An athlete may have what looks like a very mild injury and then suffer terrible consequences. The mechanism for this is thought to be loss of the ability to regulate blood flow in the brain. The brain swells when the vessels get too full of fluid. Fear of this syndrome has led to increased regulations for return to play after head injury. Treatment after traumatic brain injury is largely supportive. The best treatment focuses on assessment of the initial concussion to prevent second impact syndrome.

Since concussions may be more common in high school athletes than at the collegiate level, careful assessment has been focused on this group. The hardest part of concussion evaluation is determining the level of cognitive deficit. All doctors can look at an injured ankle and note the objective evidence of swelling, deformity, or tenderness. Since we cannot see or feel it, we do not have a quick and easy way to evaluate brain function. Different levels of education are achieved at different ages and may be affected by socioeconomic levels. It takes time to sort this out, and accurate assessment can rarely be achieved by a one-time set of questions on the sideline.

Because most athletes have a vested interest in returning to play, asking an athlete if he is confused will nearly always yield the answer "no." For this reason, objective measures have been developed to test the cognition of high school athletes and provide a scoring system. This method only works well when there is a pre-injury score for comparison. The most accurate barometer for a decline in cognition is the pre-injury cognitive level of that particular patient. Most schools do not have the resources to make this widely available. The more data we achieve with these cognitive tests, the more we can learn about cognitive decline after concussion.

Gender differences have recently become apparent in sports concussion as publicized by the media. High school girls were found to have sustained higher rates of concussion than high school boys. They also may experience different post-concussive symptoms. This makes sense with what we know about how common conditions may be affected by gender. For example, heart attack symptoms are different in women than men. However, this information flies in the face of any sports commentator who jokes that a male athlete "plays like a girl." Since most concussions are sustained during football, this was previously thought to be a problem isolated to male-dominated tackling sports. Now, we are starting to explore reasons for these gender differences. Some theorize that the increased torque on the head may be related to the weaker neck muscles in women as compared to men. Further study is necessary to quantitate and explain these differences.

One proposed mechanism for prevention of concussion is in equipment modification. Sports headgear survived great modification throughout the twentieth century. Football players started with no helmets, and then went to leather helmets. Later, fancy plastic helmets with the school logo were developed. The goal remains that more impact be absorbed by the helmet and less impact be absorbed by the head. Progress has impacted the rules of football as well as the appearance of the helmet. Players are prevented from spearing each other with the hard plastic of this helmet due to increased restrictions on the type of tackling allowed. Currently, a player may even be penalized for a missing helmet.

Since they can now fit football helmets with electronic devices, some vendors have proposed technologically advanced helmets that can assess the impact and location of the potential head injury. The data are then sent to a remote device which can alert the coach or team physician. This information could improve reporting in concussion and provide objective data on the force of the impact. The more we learn about the mechanism of concussion in sports, the more we will be able to prevent this devastating injury.

4

Diagnostic Tests

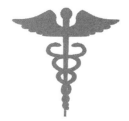

"Whenever any injury to the bone results and any fracture is suspected an xray picture should be taken at once."

—*Knute Rockne* (Rockne 1931, 11)

RADIOGRAPHY

X-rays are nearly as valuable now as they were back in the 1930s. Radiographs, also called plain films, are an accessible and easy way to view bones from the outside of your body. Professor Wilhelm Conrad Roentgen discovered that a previously unknown form of radiant energy passed through objects that regular light could not penetrate, such as his hand. We now know this form of radiant energy as X-rays. A radiograph, or X-ray picture, is formed when an electron beam is directed at a tungsten target. Radiographs used to be produced on special photographic film. Now, most radiologists use picture archiving and communications systems (PACS) to view digital images that can be shared over the Internet (Novelline 2004). This ability to see images on a computer facilitates prompt patient care. The pivotal question of "Is it broken?" can often be answered during the game rather than days after.

Currently, radiographs are a limited study since they only show the bones. Physicians utilize radiographs when a patient has an acute injury from a significant force. Since bones are pliable in children, they are more likely to suffer a fracture than a ligament or tendon injury. Since bones are stronger in adults, they are more likely to suffer a soft tissue injury than a fracture. One exception to this rule is the elderly patient population. Some patients develop osteoporosis as they age. In these patients, a very small force can cause a fracture because their bones are weak. In young children and the elderly, radiographs are a great first test to evaluate for broken bones.

Although radiographs are really helpful to look for a fracture, they provide no insight into a torn tendon or ligament. Sometimes, we can tell that a tendon is torn because the bone is slightly pushed to the wrong position on the film, but this is far more difficult to judge from a radiograph than a CT or MRI. CT was developed before MRI, and is often easier to order because it is more widely available. Also, the patient does not have to go all the way inside the machine. Even a patient with a splint can have a CT. Most emergency departments have this machine at their disposal.

CT gives a three-dimensional picture of the bones. CAT scan, which stands for computed axial tomography, is another way of referring to the same test. This test is a series of X-ray slices that allow a physician to scan through images of the patients' bones and muscles. It is almost like the patient is cut in half, so that the doctor can look directly at the area of concern. CT removes the shadows from other bones that are often found on X-rays. However, there are drawbacks to CT. If the patient has any metal parts inside, such as might occur after certain surgeries, a bright star is seen which obscures the image.

CT is great for getting a better view of certain fractures, but is not helpful for viewing muscles, intervertebral discs, or nerves. A CT can demonstrate the extent of the fracture line better than a radiograph. For example, it is really helpful to determine if a fracture goes through a joint. A fracture that goes through a joint may take longer to heal or require surgery. This is important in terms of treatment and prognosis.

MAGNETIC RESONANCE IMAGING

Magnetic resonance imaging has revolutionized the way we practice medicine. It avoids the use of ionizing radiation, which can be harmful. Remarkably, it gives a better view of the soft tissues with less radiation. MRI involves placing a patient inside a large magnet and pulsing radio waves through the body in a sequence of short bursts. Patients with metal implants, except those made of titanium or stainless steel, cannot go in the MRI because the large magnet could cause dangerous heating or movement of the metal. Cardiac pacemakers, infusion pumps, and other programmable implants cannot be used inside an MRI machine as the magnetic field can scramble the program. Because many patients hate to go inside a machine, open MRIs have been developed. Although the resolution is not as good, this is an excellent alternative to not having an MRI when it could be really helpful. The quality of the image largely depends on the power of the magnet. The higher the number of Tesla—a unit of measurement for magnetic field strength—the better we are able to view soft tissue structures.

Not only can we see the bones as in a radiograph, but also we can see ligaments, muscles, intervertebral discs, and even cartilage. Subtle changes in a bone, such as a bone bruise, that were never visualized on radiographs can be easily detected. An MRI is an instant picture of what is happening now. One way we can determine chronology on MRI is to evaluate for soft tissue swelling. If swelling is present, then the injury was relatively recent. If there is no swelling, it is far more difficult to assess the time course. This becomes important if the patient reports pain without trauma, as the time course may be necessary to theorize on the mechanism of injury. A stress fracture that does not show up on initial radiographs can be visualized on MRI. In the example shown in Figure 4.1, the patient had no fracture line on her X-rays. MRI was done and a dark fracture line is clearly apparent in the tibia.

Another exciting feature of MRI is the ability to visualize the quality of the muscle. Muscle atrophy refers to loss of muscle tone and strength. Eventually, muscle fibers are replaced with fatty or fibrotic tissue. This abnormal amount of fat or fibrosis in a muscle can be easily visualized on MRI. Even though we cannot see the nerves very well on MRI, we can easily determine which nerves have been injured by viewing the pattern of muscle atrophy. Neurogenic muscle atrophy has a different appearance than that of muscles that are simply weak from not being used. When a muscle has this appearance, the nerve that feeds the muscle is damaged. This can be seen in the MRI shown in Figure 4.2. Healthy muscle has a dark gray appearance. Atrophic muscle resembles fat. This patient had a brachial plexus injury many years before the MRI. Fatty atrophy of the deltoid is apparent on this image.

Contrast dye is used to enhance images. The dye used with MRIs is called gadolinium. This dye has received attention lately as it is thought to have a deleterious effect on the kidneys in patients with kidney disease or diabetes. As such, most doctors will recommend a blood test for kidney function prior to consideration of the dye. Typically, the dye is injected into the bloodstream to improve the picture in patients with suspected tumor or infection. These

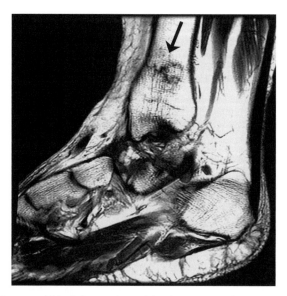

Figure 4.1. The jagged black line indicated by the arrow is the appearance of a stress fracture on MRI. This particular fracture was not apparent on radiographs alone. This is often the case with stress fractures. (Photo courtesy of the author)

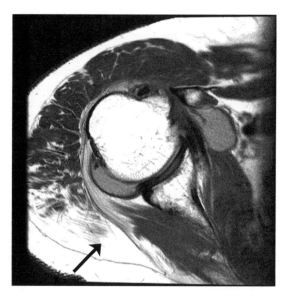

Figure 4.2. The arrow in the picture indicates an area of bright signal that typically represents fat on MRI. However, this particular area is actually the location of a shoulder muscle. This image demonstrates fatty atrophy of the muscle. (Photo courtesy of the author)

conditions demonstrate abnormally enhanced blood flow. This shows up as dye enhancement on the MRI reading. Dye is injected directly into the joint when a labral tear is suspected in the hip or shoulder. Labral tears are extremely difficult to see without the dye. If the joint is painful, the radiologist may inject some steroid or anesthetic along with the dye to provide pain relief after the procedure. If anesthetic is injected, the test is called an MR anesthetic arthrogram. It is important to note if there is any pain relief with the anesthetic. If there is pain relief, the labrum is more likely to be the source of pathology.

Some physicians argue that MRIs may be too sensitive. For example, when asymptomatic individuals are examined with an MRI, disc abnormalities can be seen in anywhere from 20 percent to 40 percent of these patients. Since these are patients who do not have back pain at the time of MRI, it is difficult to make a case for these lesions as pain generators. Some patients have severe pain with a disc abnormality, and some have no pain at all. Since pain is very subjective, we do not know if this is because the pain generator is some other structure or if some people are just more sensitive to disc pain than others.

ULTRASOUND

Also called sonography, ultrasound uses high-frequency sound waves to look inside the patient's body. Unlike the other tests we have discussed, it is difficult to visualize bone on ultrasound. Fluid appears dark because it lacks internal acoustic reflectors (Novelline 2004). Although the images are not as clear as those seen on CT or MRI, ultrasound does not have the potential to cause biologic injury. The reason for this is that it does not employ ionizing radiation. Sound waves are not harmful to even the youngest human. You may know that ultrasound is a test commonly employed to view the developing fetus. The equipment used in ultrasound is also cheaper and easier to move around, which makes it an attractive alternative to the other tests. Previously, doctors had only ordered ultrasound to view internal organs, such as the liver or kidneys. Now, we are starting to use this modality to view tendons and ligaments given its cost-effectiveness. Ultrasound is unlikely to replace radiographs when looking for a fracture, but it does have great potential to view soft tissue pathology in musculoskeletal medicine.

DEXA SCAN

Another test that may become important in the assessment of musculoskeletal injuries is the DEXA scan. This test is ordered to assess the bone density of the patient. Low bone density may be seen on radiographs, CT, or MRI as a decrease in the brightness of bone images. However, none of these tests is the best way to judge overall bone density since each was designed to assess a small part of the skeleton. The DEXA scan looks at several large bones of the body at the same time to fully assess bone quality.

DEXA stands for dual-energy x-ray absorptiometry. It becomes important when an athlete is diagnosed with a stress fracture of the insufficiency type. The test looks at bone density of the hip and the spine of the patient and compares these values to established normals. The test is reported in T- and Z-scores. The T-score compares the bone density of the patient to that of a young, healthy adult around age thirty. The Z-score compares the bone density of the patient to other patients their age and body size. The T-score is typically what we use to decide to treat patients for low bone density.

The T-score is graded in standard deviations from the mean, just like test scores that are graded on a curve. When the T-score is within 1 and 1.5 standard deviations from the mean, treatment is rarely necessary. Patients with a T-score between 1.5 and 2.5 standard deviations from the mean have osteopenia. This is not quite good enough to be normal, but not quite bad enough to be called osteoporosis. Patients with osteopenia should be on calcium and vitamin D and should be performing weight-bearing exercise at least three times a week. Patients with a T-score greater than 2.5 standard deviations from the mean have osteoporosis. There should be a high suspicion for fracture when these patients have tenderness over a bone. Patients with osteoporosis need something stronger than just supplements and weight-bearing exercise. They should be treated with a bisphosphonate or other bone-building agent. To make appropriate recommendations, it is important to know where the patient is on the spectrum of bone health.

NUCLEAR IMAGING

Nuclear imaging takes advantage of radioactive isotope metabolism throughout the body. A bone scan is a type of nuclear imaging test during which a patient is injected with a radioisotope so that areas of increased bone turnover can be viewed. The tough part of this test is the interpretation. For example, there may be increased bone turnover because of cancer, a fracture, or even arthritis. The radiologist may be able to tell which one of these diagnoses is likely by the pattern of the bone turnover. We used to use this test to diagnose stress fractures, because a stress fracture is seen on bone scan long before it is seen on radiographs. However, with advancing MRI techniques, this test is falling out of favor for diagnosis of musculoskeletal injury.

ELECTRODIAGNOSIS

Electrodiagnostic tests are the only true real-time nerve activation studies. Although usually referred to as an EMG, these tests actually consist of two parts. The first part consists of the nerve conduction studies. This series of tests utilizes the speed of an electric impulse to check for nerve injury. A small electric pulse is applied along a nerve and measured at a specified distance away, either over a muscle or the same nerve. The impulse speed is then divided by the distance it has to travel to obtain the velocity of the pulse. The speed of the impulse is measured in meters per second, similar to the miles per hour used for the speed of a car. The patient's velocity is then compared to a list of normal velocities for age and weight. This part of the test feels like when you walk across a room during the winter and get a small shock from static electricity. Most patients tolerate it fairly well. This test is very useful for diagnosing nerve injuries where there is damage to the insulating part of the nerve, resulting in a slower-moving impulse.

The name EMG or electromyography refers to the second part of the test, also called the needle exam. During this test, a tiny needle is placed into muscles of interest to look for nerve damage. The needle is similar in size to an acupuncture pin. There is a tiny microphone on the tip of the pin which magnifies sounds and creates a wave on the screen. The wave represents one motor unit, or a tiny nerve innervating one muscle fiber. The operator, also called an electromyographer, watches the screen and listens to the sound to determine if nerve damage has occurred. In general, if the motor unit wave is too large or makes abnormal sounds, there may be nerve damage. If the motor unit wave is too small, there may be muscle damage. Although the needle exam is usually the more painful part of the full test, there are rarely any complications. Sometimes, a small bruise may occur where the needle was placed. This heals in a few days and does not leave any lasting damage.

Electrodiagnostic studies are usually performed by neurologists or physiatrists. They are ordered when a patient has signs and symptoms of nerve injury. Nerve pain is usually characterized as a burning or tingling type of pain. Nerve injury presents as an area of numbness or sensory loss in the distribution of a nerve. This may be associated with weakness as well. The most widely known example of nerve injury is carpal tunnel syndrome. The carpal tunnel is the small tunnel which contains the median nerve made from the transverse carpal ligament, with tendons going through the wrist toward the fingers and the bones of the wrist. This nerve gives sensation to the thumb, index, middle, and part of the ring finger. The motor innervations include several muscles that help point the thumb toward the ceiling and a few tiny muscles that assist in bending the fingers. When a patient has carpal tunnel syndrome, he usually complains of numbness and tingling of the fingers and trouble holding on tightly with the thumb. An EMG can show if there is accompanying damage to the sensory or motor fibers of the nerve. If there is nerve damage, surgery can be helpful to release the transverse carpal ligament and make more room for the nerve in the tunnel.

5

Treatment Options

"For a bruised shoulder on the acromion process, which is generally a nerve bruise, the best treatment is hot and cold water alternately. High frequency electricity may also be used, but with caution. Rubber doughnuts on the acromion process and then covered with a sole leather padding, lifting the pad so that the weight is carried by the front and rear of the shoulder, may be successful when you have to play a man with this type of injury."

—*Knute Rockne* (Rockne 1931, 12)

TRADITIONAL TREATMENTS

The old-fashioned treatments of topical heat and ice are still useful today for most sports injuries. Unlike Rockne, we typically recommend avoiding heat for the first twenty-four to forty-eight hours. The reason for this is that heat causes blood vessels to expand. This generates more swelling around the injury and may further impair mobility. Ice is most helpful for the acute injury. Cold causes blood vessels to constrict and minimizes local swelling and bleeding into the tissues. After the acute period has passed, cold and heat can be interspersed depending on patient comfort.

The wonderful thing about topical treatments is that they don't make the patient sick to her stomach, tired, or constipated like so many of our pain medications. A few principles are important when using these treatments. Cold is best for inflammation and heat is best for spasm. Many injuries involve inflammation of the affected joint, bursa, or tendon as well as associated muscle spasm over the area. This often presents difficulty in choosing the appropriate agent. Rockne may be right; they may work well together.

Since heat tends to loosen stiffness, heat may be best before activity. Ice tends to calm down an overworked area, and may be best utilized after activity. This is not a strict guideline, but gives patients a framework to try out which treatment works best for them. Heat comes in several forms. The most common form is the heating pad that can be microwaved or plugged into the wall. There are also topical heating pad patches available. Generally, topical heat that dissipates after twenty minutes is the safest form. It is fairly easy to get a burn with a topical heat source that remains at the same strength if it is left against the skin for more than thirty minutes. Pain in an area often alters the ability to sense the burn. In fact, heating pad burns are so common there is even a name given to the appearance of the skin after a burn from the heating pad. This is called erythema ab igne.

In contrast, skin damage from aggressive ice application is rather rare in patients with normal sensation. This can be an issue for patients with nerve damage. When heat or cold is about to damage the skin, our sensory receptors feel pain and send this message back to the brain by way of the peripheral nerves. If there is a disconnect in this system, the signal does not get back. Patients with sensory loss should be carefully monitored for color changes of the skin during application of heat or ice. Generally, applying a cloth between the ice and the skin and leaving the ice on for no longer than twenty minutes will be well within the margin of safety.

There is one exception to this rule. Ice should not be directly applied over an area where a nerve is superficial. Two areas of concern are the medial elbow for the ulnar nerve and the lateral knee for the peroneal nerve. Ice, especially when used together with compression, may cause local ischemia to the nerve and decrease its ability to function. In the elbow, this could result in decreased grip strength. In the knee, this could result in foot drop. Both conditions will likely be self-limited, but may be best avoided.

Electric stimulation is another topical pain treatment surprisingly recommended by Rockne that we still use today. This involves the application of adhesive electrode pads to the body in the area of pain by a physical therapist. This is thought to work for pain relief by stimulating the nerves so they do not send the pain signal back to the brain. Another added benefit is that it may stimulate chemicals in the body that decrease local pain. Treatments usually last twenty to thirty minutes. They are gradually decreased as the pain improves. If the pain does not improve but the patient gets relief from the treatments, a home unit can be dispensed with instruction so that the patient can perform these treatments independently. Usually, pain from muscle strain improves and this is not necessary. However, the low back is one area where pain may persist, and medications have significant limitations. I have found transcutaneous electric nerve stimulation to be particularly helpful in patients with low back pain given its low side effect profile and its use in conjunction with physical therapy.

Compression or splinting of the injured part plays a key role in return to athletic activity after injury. The injured limb should be immobilized in the position of function. The reason for this is to prevent contracture and decrease edema. As more collagen is laid down to heal the injured part, this scar tissue may cause restricted motion of the surrounding tissues. The patient is positioned in a splint such that even if contracture or effusion occurs, it will have the least impact.

For the ankle joint, this position is with the ankle at a ninety degree angle or in the dorsiflexed position. This position is also the close-packed position of the joint. This means that it is the position in which the least space is available for swelling at the joint. If there is no room for the swelling, the amount of fluid that escapes into the tissues will likely be decreased. This principle of positioning the limb in such a way as to prevent the complications of post-injury scar tissue and minimize effusion can be applied to other joints as well. Contracture prevention is of particular importance in the shoulder. Patients who suffer from this complication may not be able to perform such simple tasks as brushing their teeth or combing their hair.

The type of splint applied depends on the extent and location of the injury. Prefabricated or off-the-shelf splints are usually readily available and can be easily removed and applied. Unfortunately, they do not often fit patients who are very large or small. Custom-molded splints are best used in these cases, but they take longer to make and may be more expensive for the patient. Casting is reserved for fracture management or post-operative positioning after certain tendon procedures. Although a cast provides excellent immobilization, it cannot be adjusted to allow for edema and it cannot be removed to assess the sensation of the injured part. Typically, casts are utilized in patients who will require a longer period of intense immobilization.

There are many devices available for protected weight-bearing. Typically, these devices utilize the upper body to provide additional support for an injured lower limb. Crutches are the most commonly used assistive devices in lower-limb injury. Crutches should be adjusted to the height of the injured athlete and appropriately padded so as to avoid nerve injury at the shoulder or the hand. If the patient has sustained concurrent upper- and lower-limb injuries, platform crutches or walkers are available. These allow the patient to rest their elbows on the device and bear weight through the forearms. Even older athletes usually despise the thought of a walker, but this may be the only alternative to a wheelchair in patients with decreased upper-body strength or injuries of multiple limbs.

Patients with musculoskeletal injury used to be hospitalized and prescribed weeks of bed rest. Now, we know that the more patients move around, the better the outcome. This is likely related to increased circulation of blood that occurs with walking as well as avoidance of the complications of immobility. Prolonged bed rest contributes to decreased pulmonary function and increased lower-limb swelling. Blood clots, bladder problems, and constipation occur in patients who are prevented from moving around. Frequent complications prolong the course of musculoskeletal injury.

Atrophy of muscle tissue begins two weeks after nerve injury or lack of use. This may be even more dangerous in those with underlying bone injury. We have learned that bone heals best when the muscles and nerves surrounding the injury are kept as healthy as possible. Exercising the muscle also mobilizes soft tissue edema and improves mood. Early range of motion exercises prevent joint contracture.

Unlike prolonged immobilization, elevation of the injured part is still helpful in treatment of musculoskeletal injury. This is usually accomplished by propping the injured limb on pillows. Elevation works well in conjunction with ice application. Blood tends to pool at the lowest point of the body. If a patient is lying in bed with the lower limb propped up, the lowest point is actually the buttocks. This is why hospitalized patients are routinely checked for skin break down on their buttocks.

The pain medications section at the drug store seems to be growing with the increasing age of the population and the availability of a wide variety of sports for athletes of all ages. Anti-inflammatories remain a popular choice for pain in both the over-the-counter and prescribed formulations. This class does not include acetaminophen, which has only a weak anti-inflammatory effect. This medication functions more as an analgesic (painkiller) and antipyretic (fever reducer). Ibuprofen and naproxen are the most popular over-the-counter anti-inflammatory medications. Ibuprofen is taken three to six times a day and naproxen is only taken twice. Both medications work in a similar way to reduce inflammation by interfering with the cellular pathway that signals prostaglandins.

Injured tissue sends out cells to signal the injury to the body. These signal cells trigger the immune response, which involves prostaglandins. This response can be helpful to our body in that there is an internal mechanism for tissue repair. Unfortunately, the process is painful. Nonsteroidal anti-inflammatory medications work by blocking the part of this complicated pathway that signals the feeling of pain. Some patients worry that this will block all of the healing effects of the pathway. This is not the case. Pharmacology has become so selective that we are able to further limit the action of these medications to selectively target pain mediators with fewer side effects.

Selective COX-2 inhibitors were developed for this reason. COX stands for cyclooxygenase, an enzyme that functions in this biochemical pathway. Prostaglandins in the body trigger pain, but they also protect the stomach. These medications were formulated for patients who cannot tolerate the potential adverse effects of nonselective anti-inflammatories on the stomach lining. Initially, changes in the stomach lining may result in pain. Later, an ulcer may form. Ulcers are particularly dangerous because they are a source of internal bleeding. Some prescribers were able to circumvent these risks by prescribing a medication along with the anti-inflammatory to protect the stomach. However, most patients do not like to take two medications when one may do the job. Selective COX-2 inhibitors are theoretically able to block the unpleasant inflammatory effects of pain and swelling without the deleterious effect on the protective lining of the stomach.

Concern over gastric ulcers in those who use anti-inflammatories led to great excitement over the release of these selective COX-2 inhibitors at the end of the twentieth century. Celecoxib was the first of these agents to be approved by the FDA in December 1998. Rofecoxib followed in May 1999. Increased use of these agents led to the discovery that they cause cardiovascular side effects, perhaps by the mechanism of increased blood pressure. In a very interesting phenomenon of pharmacology, we learned more about all of the anti-inflammatories after the well-publicized removal of rofecoxib from the market in 2004. All anti-inflammatories, even the over-the-counter ones, may cause high blood pressure to varying degrees. The difficult factor in the study of these medications is that pain may cause hypertension as well. Acutely, hypertension becomes dangerous in regard to the increased likelihood of heart attack or stroke. It is best that patients who have cardiovascular risks avoid anti-inflammatories.

Another concern with all anti-inflammatories is possible adverse renal effects. In the recommended dosage, these medications do not typically incite kidney problems in those with no history. However, in those with previously known kidney problems or in higher than the recommended dosage, these medications have long been implicated in decreased renal function. Normal kidneys can often recover from an impairment function with discontinuation of the offending agent and consistent rehydration. Diseased kidneys have a much more difficult and protracted recovery from an insult. As such, anti-inflammatories are not used in patients with kidney disease.

Avoidance of anti-inflammatories is nearly impossible, as they are highly recommended in every musculoskeletal condition except fracture management. The safest and most widely recommended option is acetaminophen. This is available over-the-counter. Acetaminophen may have mild renal effects, but these are not typically found in patients who abide by the recommended dosage of no more than 4,000 milligrams in a twenty-four-hour period. The liver is the organ we are most concerned about with acetaminophen use. Regular use can elevate the liver enzymes. Levels often return to normal after discontinuation. Long-term sequelae may develop in patients with known liver disease who use acetaminophen; therefore, it is best avoided in these patients. Unfortunately, anti-inflammatories also cannot be used in patients with liver disease as these patients carry an increased risk for gastrointestinal bleeding.

Another group of medications that has come into favor is neuropathic pain medications. Neuropathic pain refers to pain from nerve irritation or injury and has a tingling or burning quality. The most popular of these is gabapentin. This medication was discovered as a medication to prevent seizures. Since it was found to decrease pain signals as well, it is now used for neuropathic pain. It works on the calcium channels in the nerves to decrease pain signals. Unfortunately, it also makes patients tired, may cause dizziness or swelling, and may affect the patient's mood. The feelings of fatigue tend to improve with increased use of the medication. Recommendations to prevent fatigue include taking the medication before bedtime, starting on the lowest effective dose, and increasing the dose slowly as the side effects wear off.

Other neuropathic pain medications include amitriptyline, nortriptyline, and pregabalin. Amitriptyline and nortriptyline come from as class of medications known as tricyclic antidepressants. These medications have been around a long time to treat depression. At lower doses, they can be helpful for neuropathic pain. They work on neurotransmitters in the brain and sodium channels in the nerves. Common side effects include dry mouth, urinary retention, weight gain, and somnolence. Citrus flavors from hard candy or juice can be helpful for dry mouth.

Pregabalin works on calcium channels in the central nervous system and also functions as an anti-seizure medication. As such, it carries a similar side effect profile to gabapentin. Unlike gabapentin, it also has the indication for fibromyalgia. Fibromyalgia is a condition in which the patient is sensitive to pain at soft tissue trigger points throughout the body, but does not carry the diagnosis of systemic rheumatic disease. Similar to neurontin, pregabalin should be started at lower doses and titrated up to minimize side effects.

Stronger pain medications exist, but these may be best reserved for severe traumatic injury, post-operative pain, or patients with chronic illness who cannot have anti-inflammatories. Opioids are generally regarded as the strongest pain medications due to their ability to create dangerous levels of somnolence in patients. Commonly prescribed opioids are oxycodone, hydrocodone, and morphine. Opioids work on receptors in the brain to induce relaxation. Common adverse effects include nausea, vomiting, constipation, urinary retention, and even addiction. Prescribers are most concerned about addiction. These medications tend to make patients feel better, but they may not have any favorable effects on the outcome of musculoskeletal injury. As such, they are best provided in a limited supply with patient education on the projected time course of their use.

One way to get around the risks of oral pain medications is to look for effective topical medications. Topical medications are applied to the skin in the form of a gel, cream, or a patch. The hope is that these agents will work at the site of injury without causing problems for other parts of the body. Although minimal systemic absorption has been reported with these agents, the possibility still exists. The most tragic case of known side effects from topical pain medications occurred in the summer of 2007.

Salicylic acid toxicity was reported as the cause of death in a young female runner. This is the active ingredient in aspirin, but the patient was not taking any oral medications. She was applying topical Bengay and using Bengay patches as well as another un-named over-the-counter topical agent. Salicylic acid is the active ingredient in many of the commercially available pain relief creams and lotions. Prior to this incident, it was considered very safe in its topical form. Cases like this illustrate that we may not know the threshold for when a locally applied medication spreads to the bloodstream. These medications can certainly be helpful for musculoskeletal pain with a limited side effect profile. However, they must be applied according to the package directions. The skin where the agent has been applied should not be occluded but left open to air or loose clothing.

Prescription topical pain medications are also available. Capsaicin and lidoderm are both applied to the skin, but work in very different ways. Although capsaicin burns like Bengay, it does not work in the same fashion. The burning feeling comes from the ingredient that the medication is derived from in hot peppers. The medication works on a chemical in the body called substance P. The capsaicin depletes the local supply of substance P in the nerve endings, which disrupts the transport of the pain signal to the brain. Due to its burning action, this can only be applied to intact skin. Patients should wear gloves when applying and avoid touching their eyes after using this medication. It can be helpful for both local muscle pain and neuropathic pain. It is likely best avoided in acute injury as skin laceration or bruising may be present.

The newest class of prescription topical pain medication patches in the United States is a topical anti-inflammatory. Although we have been using topical steroids for skin conditions and for iontophoresis for years, the only topical anti-inflammatory that we had available was the over-the- counter aspirin analog in Bengay and related products. Topical diclofenac was approved by the U.S. Food and Drug Administration in 2007. This medication has been around in its oral form for years, but the patches were developed for local application to reduce systemic side effects. The patches still carry the black box warning about possible cardiovascular side effects like their oral counterparts. Limited studies have suggested that side effects, especially gastro-intestinal side effects, may be less frequent with the topical form.

Steroids are the strongest anti-inflammatory medications that we have in our armamentarium. Corticosteroids, or sugar steroids, are the type of steroids that help decrease inflammation. They can be taken orally, applied topically, or injected directly at the site of pain. The most commonly prescribed form of oral steroids is a steroid taper. This is a previously determined dosing of ste-roids that starts with the highest dose and ends with the lowest dose. The rea-son for the tapering is that the adrenal glands in the body make sugar steroids. If oral steroids are ingested at a consistently high dose, this can signal the body to stop making its own steroids. Gradually decreasing the dose avoids suppres-sion of the adrenal glands.

Sugar steroids function in the body's response to pain, inflammation, and infection. Modifying this response may result in unpleasant side effects. Possi-ble side effects with oral steroids include gastrointestinal ulcers, increases in blood sugar levels, hunger, mood elevation, fluid retention, and a possible decrease in the body's ability to fight off infection. The risk of gastrointestinal ulcers is similar to the risk in other anti-inflammatories, but may be slightly higher. Most patients will not notice the elevated blood sugar levels, but this can be of particular concern in diabetes. Hunger, mood elevation, and fluid retention are generally self-limited and well tolerated. If the patient is already ill, steroids are a bad idea because they can worsen the illness. Most patients who are not infected do not get an infection from taking steroids. This tends to be more of an issue in patients who are already sick.

Topical steroids can be applied in the form of creams or lotions or pulsed into the skin with electric waves as in iontophoresis. Most of the creams and lotions just work on the layers of skin. These are great medications for skin conditions like psoriasis, but they are not likely to decrease musculoskeletal pain. If steroids are applied with the heat of electricity as in iontophoresis or ultrasound waves as in phonophoresis, they tend to be effective for pain with very minimal side effects. One reason we know that these treatments are unlikely to have systemic adverse effects is that animal studies have shown that the steroids do not actually penetrate the layers of skin during this procedure. This certainly makes it difficult to explain their efficacy. Perhaps, patients get additional relief from the heat treatments with the steroid medium that is attributed to an anti-inflammatory effect. Regardless, iontophoresis and phonophoresis can be safe and effective alternatives for patients who cannot take steroids.

Injected steroids usually avoid any potential gastrointestinal risks, but they are not without complications. Although very low, there is still a theoretical risk of infection. Proper cleansing of the skin with bactericidal solution has greatly reduced this risk. Injections should be avoided in any patients who have a known infection. Pain and bleeding at the injection site usually occur. These do not last very long and often the benefit of pain relief outweighs these risks. Injection directly into a nerve may result in temporary sensory or motor impairment. Injections should never be performed close to the known course of a large nerve. Injection directly into a tendon may weaken the tendon. This is of particular concern in the Achilles, which may be prone to rupture from cortisone injections.

Most doctors recommend no more than four cortisone injections per year. Like all recommendations, there may be some patients who have no problem with five, six, or seven cortisone injections. This is simply the estimated threshold limit before we think that the cortisone causes degeneration of the tendon or bone metabolism problems. In regard to bone metabolism, corticosteroids have been implicated as a cause of osteoporosis and avascular necrosis. These disorders are unusual with one or two injections, but may factor into the decision to try an injection in patients with a known bone metabolism problem.

Diabetes is the most common cause of neuropathy in the United States. Patients with diabetes need to be aware of how steroid injections may act differently on their bodies because of the disease. Diabetes can induce neuropathic pain that is similar in quality and location to mechanical compression of a nerve. When patients have both diabetes and mechanical nerve compression, the cause of the pain may not be obvious. Steroid injections for nerve pain may not be effective if the pain is from diabetic neuropathy. Since injected steroids may temporarily increase blood sugar, this can cause an adverse effect on the diabetes with little benefit for nerve pain. Most patients with diabetes do very well with steroid injections at the bursa or the joint, but caution should be exercised in nerve injections for this patient population.

Pain medication can help with comfort after injury, but compliance with physical therapy is usually the real reason behind improvement in musculo-skeletal injury. Current outpatient insurance benefits cover two weekly visits for eight to twelve weeks of physical therapy. There may be a co-payment, but most insurance companies will cover therapy. Given the increasing body of knowledge about the benefits of exercise for overall health, some insurance companies are now even giving discounts for gym memberships. Most physical therapists can devise a home program that the patient can continue at their own local gym when her therapy has ended.

The goals of physical therapy vary widely with the variation in forms of musculoskeletal injury. Initial goals involve decreasing pain and swelling and increasing range of motion. As pain improves, therapy shifts to focus on cor-recting underlying muscle imbalances and strengthening the area around the injured part. Later, therapy may focus on sport-specific drills to simulate ath-letic activities in a noncontact situation. Once the athlete can perform these drills without pain or instability, they can return to game play.

COMPLEMENTARY AND ALTERNATIVE MEDICINE

With so many known side effects of traditional pharmaceutical agents, it is no surprise that patients have turned to nutritional supplements in the treat-ment of musculoskeletal injury. Unfortunately, there is limited regulation of these agents by the Food and Drug Administration. The term nutraceuticals is now used commonly to describe a food product or its ingredients that could be used for medicinal properties. Debate continues regarding whether foods con-sumed as part of a balanced diet could be nutraceuticals. For example, ginger remains in both the food and drug categories. Ginger is often served with sushi as a popular entrée. However, some patients get relief of nausea or motion sickness from this food or medication.

The most widely promoted nutraceuticals in the media, glucosamine and chondroitin, share an oceanic origin. Glucosamine, a derivative of shellfish chitin, specifically targets cartilage. Chondroitin is thought to have a weak anti-inflammatory effect. The most notable trial to date for glucosamine and chondroitin is the National Institutes of Health-funded GAIT (Glucosamine/ chondroitin Arthritis Intervention trial) involving over 1,500 patients. Involved subjects with knee osteoarthritis were followed for nearly six months for a decrease in knee pain. Patients took a daily dose of 1500 milligrams of glucosamine, 1200 milligrams of chondroitin sulfate, both glucosamine and chondroitin sulfate, 200 milligrams of celecoxib, or placebo. Celecoxib is a selective COX-2 inhibitor. Overall, glucosamine and chondroitin alone or together did not demonstrate pain relief in a significant number of the participants. However, when the data from the subgroup of patients with the most severe pain was analyzed separately, it did appear that the combination of glucosamine and chondroitin may have a significant benefit in pain reduction.

Regardless of the efficacy of glucosamine and chondroitin, these agents rarely cause adverse effects. Since glucosamine is an aminomonosaccharide, there has been concern about the role of its sugar constituent in diabetic patients. Limited studies have shown no increase in blood sugar levels in normal patients and no worsening of disease in diabetics. There has been less speculation about chemical side effects of chondroitin. Regardless, there have been no documented adverse effects on the chemistry of the blood or urine in randomized controlled trials. Current doses recommended as safe for patients are up to 2000 milligrams per day for glucosamine and 1200 milligrams for chondroitin sulfate. The best evidence we have is that the combination is unlikely to cause harm and may decrease pain in patients with moderate to severe knee osteoarthritis.

Avocado soybean unsaponifiables have received attention for their anabolic and anti-inflammatory effects on cartilage. They are made from natural ingredients found in avocado and soybeans and thought to decrease cartilage breakdown or prevent arthritis. In humans, there was no additional efficacy with doses higher than 300 milligrams. Side effects were similar to those of placebo. Three placebo-controlled trials with the 300-milligram dose for three to six months led to a significant improvement in functional activity and reduced analgesic requirement. In one of these studies, patients showed continued improvement in outcomes after a two-month follow-up period of no treatment. Overall, patients with hip osteoarthritis reported better outcomes than those with knee osteoarthritis. Further studies have refuted these initial claims of efficacy. Regardless, since these are naturally occurring foods, it is difficult to recommend against them.

Most patients are aware of the benefits of the omega-3 fatty acids in fish oil for cardiovascular and inflammatory diseases. Omega-3 polyunsaturated fatty acids, such as linolenic acid and eicosapentenoic acid (EPA), have been investigated for osteoarthritis as well. Like avocado soybean saponifiables, early studies were promising. Although fish oil is of benefit in patients with rheumatoid arthritis, there does not appear to be a similar clinical benefit in osteoarthritis patients. Given the helpful cardiovascular and anti-inflammatory effects, it is certainly worth taking these agents. Since they have blood-thinning properties, patients may be cautioned to stop taking these supplements prior to surgical procedures. A recent review of the cardiology literature suggests that there is no greater risk of bleeding when taking omega-3 fatty acids, even in combination with coumadin or aspirin. *Consumer Reports* recommends choosing a fish oil brand mainly on price. Their tests of the leading brands for contamination with mercury, dioxin-dioxin-like PCBs, and decomposition were negative. All sixteen brands tested contained as much omega-3s (as EPA and DHA) as their labels promised. Freezing the capsules was recommended to prevent potential side effects such as bloating, gas, and a "fishy" taste.

Minerals have also been advertised for the treatment of osteoarthritis. Selenium, boron, and zinc may decrease the incidence of osteoarthritis. Like omega-3 fatty acids, selenium has proven anti-inflammatory effects. Unfortunately, critical review of studies involving selenium alone or in combination with vitamins A, C, and E failed to show clinical benefit. Boron is present in nearly twice the concentration in healthy as compared to arthritic femur heads. Areas of the world where people consume more boron (3 milligrams to 10 milligrams as compared to 1 milligram or less) have a lower incidence of arthritis. Twenty subjects demonstrated decreased symptoms of osteoarthritis when taking 6 milligrams of boron daily.

Patients with osteoarthritis exhibited higher serum copper levels and lower serum zinc levels than controls in one study of serum samples. Since low zinc may be associated with osteoarthritis, some companies market zinc as a way to prevent osteoarthritis. There are no clear data to support this. Although copper levels appear to be elevated in osteoarthritis, it is sold as a dietary supplement. There is no role for this agent for osteoarthritis treatment, other than the potential to aggravate the problem. Mineral toxicity can be a significant issue. High doses of zinc not only cause zinc toxicity, but also yield subsequent copper deficiency. This may result in significant problems with the cardiovascular system and the red blood cells.

Vitamins A, C, and E have received attention for their antioxidant properties. Vitamin A in the human body is derived from consumption of beta-carotene, one of the naturally occurring carotenoids. Studies have shown both benefit and harm in osteoarthritis. The reason for this may be that different carotenoids have different effects. Carotenoids are converted to vitamin A in the body. As a fat-soluble vitamin, vitamin A has received attention for its potential negative effects. Carotenoids have not been fully explored in terms of toxicity, but editorials in the ophthalmologic literature express concern over this possibility. Remarkably, lutein is sold on the Internet together with zeaxanthin. There are data for this combination in promotion of ocular health.

Since one of these agents is associated with a lower likelihood of osteoarthritis and the other is associated with a higher likelihood, it makes sense to avoid this dietary supplement altogether unless used for the prevention of macular degeneration.

Vitamin C may reduce pain in hip and knee osteoarthritis. The Framingham cohort study found that intake of 120 to 200 milligrams of vitamin C daily resulted not only in decreased knee pain but also in a much lower risk of osteoarthritis progression (McAlindon 1996). Given the large number of patients involved in this study, vitamin C became a promising arthritis treatment in the mid-1990s. Eight years later, further analysis in the guinea pig model of osteoarthritis called these results into question. In animal studies, vitamin C appeared to actually worsen osteoarthritis. Although vitamin C has an effect in osteoarthritis, further study is necessary to determine whether this effect is positive or negative in humans. As a water-soluble vitamin, toxicity is less likely to occur with oral ingestion. Unlike other vitamins, the only reported side effect is diarrhea. Since vitamin C certainly has other favorable effects in the body and very low side effects, it is certainly worth trying for osteoarthritis.

Vitamin E appears to play a smaller role in osteoarthritis than vitamin C. The most promising clinical data on vitamin E come from the Framingham cohort study. Men who had a higher dietary intake of vitamin E were less likely to have progression of osteoarthritis. Vitamin E did not affect the incidence of osteoarthritis. Currently, there is little evidence to recommend vitamin E for osteoarthritis treatment. However, Vitamin E is often recommended for its role in healthy skin.

A clear player in bone metabolism, increased doses of vitamin D are recommended for women with osteoporosis. They may be helpful for those with osteoarthritis as well. Women with low vitamin D levels were found to have a greater risk of radiographic progression of osteoarthritis in two studies. Since those who are older are more likely to have osteoarthritis, osteoporosis, and lower vitamin D levels, it is hard to sort out the possible confounding factors. Proper dosing may require a serum level. Fortunately, toxicity of vitamin D is rare. This occurs at consistent daily doses greater than or equal to 40,000 IU daily.

The current controversy surrounding vitamin D applies to the type of vitamin D prescribed. Vitamin D2, ergocalciferol, is more widely available by prescription in the United States. However, vitamin D3, cholecalciferol, is more bioavailable. The biggest concern is not so much the type of vitamin D, but that low levels are appropriately treated. Current recommendations include checking a 25-OH vitamin D level in high-risk patients, such as women with dark skin pigment, lack of sun exposure, disorders of gastrointestinal absorption, prior stress fracture, or age greater than sixty-five. If the level of vitamin D in the bloodstream is below 30 nanograms per milliliter, then the patient should be treated with eight weeks of ergocalciferol at 50,000 units per week. If there is concern for decreased gastrointestinal absorption, the serum level can be repeated at the end of the eight weeks to monitor for treatment efficacy.

Europeans commonly use willow bark, a natural source of salicylic acid, to treat musculoskeletal pain. There is one trial comparing willow bark with placebo for hip and knee osteoarthritis. A dose of willow bark containing 240 milligrams of salicin did decrease pain in the seventy-eight subjects. This botanical extract was well tolerated. A trial for low back pain compared willow bark in the same dose with rofecoxib and found similar pain reduction and adverse effects after four weeks. Although this study was not for osteoarthritis treatment, it addressed the potential negative effects and the cost difference between the two agents. Rofecoxib, a prescription anti-inflammatory, was 40 percent more expensive. Trials of longer duration are needed to address the efficacy of willow bark for osteoarthritis.

Commercially available willow bark is derived most commonly from the white willow, but can come from the crack willow, purple willow, and violet willow. It is listed in the German Commission E of approved herbs in terms of safety and efficacy with the indication of analgesia. Little is known about the long-term use of this agent in the United States. Critics suggest avoiding its use in children to avoid the risk of Reye's syndrome, which may occur when children are treated with aspirin after the chicken pox or another viral illness. Aspirin has a similar chemical structure to willow bark. Patients with a history of aspirin allergy, peptic ulcer disease, or renal disease should avoid this agent.

Although the negative effects of nutraceuticals are not widely known, they have been less harmful when compared to nonsteroidal anti-inflammatory drugs (NSAIDS) in animal and human studies. Often, they can be tolerated for a longer period than NSAIDs. Most are less expensive on a monthly basis. The cost difference may be negligible when comparing the duration needed to achieve pain relief. It is important to inform your physician if you are taking nutraceuticals. Unfortunately, we have far less hard medical data to stand behind these agents, but we continue to become more familiar with potential drug interactions and adverse effects.

Complementary and alternative medicine treatments have become increasingly popular in recent years due to their low side effect profile. Some would argue that this increased acceptance of alternative therapies is related to inadequacies in the approach to pain taken by traditional medicine. Regardless, utilization of massage, acupuncture, and chiropractic treatment appears to be on the rise. Although massage is a popular activity at many modern day spas, this medical treatment actually dates back to Hippocrates who lived in ancient Greece before Galen, the team physician to the gladiators mentioned in Chapter 1. It is difficult to dispute that rubbing the injured part feels good, and has felt good to patients for thousands of years. Massage can provide pain relief and fluid mobilization. Unfortunately, this effect may not last as long as the pain.

Acupuncture involves placing needles in the skin in areas designed for healing. There is a component of healing energy and Eastern medicine involved in acupuncture. Studies have the most unbiased outcome when subjects are randomly assigned to different treatments. It is incredibly difficult to fake acupuncture. The patient is either getting pins stuck into them or not. As such, it is tough to reliably compare acupuncture with a placebo treatment. Regardless, there are good data for pain relief with acupuncture. Reliable data for relief of medical conditions such as stroke and diabetes with acupuncture are currently lacking.

Chiropractic treatment varies widely with the practitioner. Many chiropractors perform spinal manipulation. This is safe and can provide relief in a selected population. We recommend that patients with acute disc herniation avoid aggressive spinal manipulation until their condition has improved. Patients over age sixty-five, those with a family history of stroke, and patients with rheumatoid arthritis should avoid aggressive neck manipulation. In general, treatments such as gentle traction and application of electric stimulation are safe when performed by a trained professional.

ERGONOMICS

Patients frequently ask about the best furniture products to relieve pain in musculoskeletal injury. Although advertisers would have you believe otherwise, this is no simple issue. As you can imagine, most patients will not continue to sleep in an uncomfortable bed. Limited availability of good data makes it hard to recommend one mattress over another. There is one randomized study done in Europe which reports that a medium firm mattress may decrease back pain. However, medium firm may mean a lot of things to a lot of different manufacturers. In general, trial and error is best to find the most comfortable sleeping surface.

Athletes with back pain usually feel the best in a side-lying position with a pillow between the legs. If there is a disc herniation present, it may be better to sleep with the painful side toward the ceiling and the non-painful limb against the bed. Theoretically, this will prevent gravity from further encouraging the disc toward the nerve during sleep. Patients with neck pain feel best with a small pillow that does not flex or extend the neck to extremes. Some patients substitute a small towel roll for a pillow or wear a soft neck collar to bed. Patients with limb injuries should elevate the affected extremity while sleeping. During the night, patients with nerve injuries should avoid pressure on common areas of compression, such as the medial elbow and the lateral knee.

Office furniture provides another recommendation dilemma due to lack of unbiased information. In general, keeping the computer at eye level and the hips and knees at ninety degrees is best for most ailments. Use of a headset in lieu of a phone receiver can be incredibly helpful for neck pain. Patients with pain in the neck and back should get up from their desks and perform light stretching whenever possible. Most of us carry our stress in our neck muscles, and we live in a very stressful society. A simple break from prolonged positioning can take some strain out of the neck muscles during the day when the patient cannot access the gym.

6

Prevention

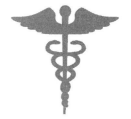

"A player who is injured should not be put back too soon. This may cause a recurrence of the same injury sufficient enough to keep the man out for the season."

—*Knute Rockne* (Rockne 1931, 12)

M ost athletes desire to return to play as quickly as possible. The obvious danger is an injury that is even worse than the initial insult. The stakes are typically highest for head injury, but even limb injuries can weaken reaction times and put athletes in a dangerous situation. Prior to returning to a game situation, athletes should demonstrate pain-free range of motion. At the very least, strength should be normal. Insensate parts should be well protected. The athlete should be able to demonstrate participation in sport-specific drills without instability.

Proprioceptive deficits may contribute to rates of re-injury. This is especially true in cases of ankle and knee sprain. Proprioception is the ability of the mind to sense the limb's position in space. Examples of proprioceptive exercises include trying to balance on a wobble board or ankle disc for recovery after ankle sprain or performing squats with the eyes closed for recovery after knee sprain. Careful practice of proprioceptive exercises enhances balance and may even improve sports performance.

BRACING

In some joints, bracing is effective for both treatment and prevention of injury. Ankle braces help to improve mobility and decrease swelling in the acute period after injury. Since the ligaments are stretched in even the mild form of ankle sprain, there is a tendency for the ankle to roll. Ankle braces prevent inversion injury of the ankle during sports activity. Lace-up ankle braces with medial and lateral stays to prevent twisting the ankle are commercially available and prevent further injury. They do not need to be worn during daily activities, but should be worn in athletes with a history of ankle sprain.

Bracing plays a controversial role in the prevention of knee ligamentous injuries. Knee bracing can be helpful for mobility, pain relief, and swelling in the acute period. Patellar tracking braces may even have a role in chronic knee pain. However, bracing is not recommended for prevention of knee ligamentous injuries. The reason for this is that there are conflicting data as to whether knee bracing causes or prevents injury. The reason for the controversy may be related to the complex action of the knee joint. Although we think of the knee joint as a hinge that just allows flexion and extension, there is a fair amount of sideways motion in the knee. Ankle sprain nearly always results from inversion injury at the ankle. Knee sprain can happen from any one of a variety of mechanisms, the most frequent of which is a pivot-type movement. For now, we do not recommend prophylactic knee bracing.

There is little information about bracing for prevention of upper-limb injury. Wrist braces can be helpful for the treatment of carpal tunnel syndrome by maintaining the wrist in neutral. Elbow braces can be helpful for symptomatic relief of pain over the lateral elbow. Custom elbow extension splints can prevent compression of the ulnar nerve as it winds around the elbow. Shoulder braces can help maintain the shoulder in a position of function while the patient is healing from surgery. Currently, there is no evidence to suggest that any of these braces would prevent injury.

STRETCHING

Stretching is an important part of any exercise regimen for injury prevention and performance enhancement. In regard to injury prevention, flexible muscles withstand impact better due to the elastic properties of muscle. There is little debate among health care practitioners about the merits of stretching for injury prevention. In fact, stretching is a key component of most physical therapy treatment plans. The controversy relates to performance enhancement and the type of stretching.

Recent media attention publicized the difference between static and dynamic stretching for performance enhancement. Static stretching is the more commonly known form of stretching. An example of static stretching is sitting on the ground with the legs apart while reaching for the toes in a slow controlled action. We used to tell patients to make sure not to bounce during this motion. Actually, dynamic stretching involves a little of this bouncing. An example of dynamic stretching is marching in place or performing high kicks. Studies have recently shown that static stretching prior to a workout may decrease performance during the workout. Dynamic stretching before a workout may increase muscle power during the workout.

Although dynamic stretching may be the best way to shine in the game, this does not discount a potential role of static stretching. Perhaps, this type of stretching is best performed after a workout, when the muscles are already warm. Static stretching is certainly beneficial in weekend warriors suffering from overuse injuries. Plantar fasciitis responds well to continued stretching of the bottom of the foot. Treatment of lateral epicondylitis employs stretching of the wrist extensors. Iliotibial band syndrome does not improve without consistent stretching of the soft tissue of the lateral hip.

7

Current and Future Research

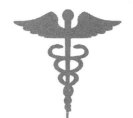

"A team should never be coddled in regard to their physical ailments, but rather should be made to adopt a Spartan attitude. Every man should report any injury, so as to make sure that a more serious injury may not follow and also to make sure that no man who should not play is allowed to get into a game or scrimmage. No man should ever be played if he has an ailment of a chronic type, as playing a rough game such as football is, might very easily give him a permanent injury."

—*Knute Rockne* (Rockne 1931, 12)

ERGOGENIC AIDS

Performance enhancement may be even more important to the athlete than injury prevention. As in any discipline, the best way to excel at sport is consistent practice. Since results from practice are consistently slow and may reach a plateau, research focuses on modification of factors that enhance performance. Medical researchers struggle to find the right levels of protein, fat, and sugar to maximize output from the human body.

Debate continues about what foods to eat and at what times of the day to achieve the fastest running time or the longest jump. We do know for sure that protein is necessary to build muscle. The amount of protein required is based on the weight of the individual. The recommended dietary intake of protein is 0.8 grams per kilogram of body weight per day. Athletes in training typically need twice this amount, in range from 1.6 grams to 1.8 grams per kilogram of body weight daily. Eating more protein than the recommended amount does not increase the benefits of protein. Protein is filtered by the kidneys. Consequently, concern has been raised about impairment of kidney function with increased ingestion of protein. Intake under 2.8 grams per kilogram of body weight does not impair renal function.

Sugar is necessary for power performance. When the blood sugar gets too low, the athlete gets lethargic. The body usually takes care of this by breaking down body fat to release stored sugar. This process can go wrong in athletes with low body fat that do not snack consistently. In general, complex carbohydrates may be better for endurance activities since they last longer in the blood. Fat is not necessary to ingest since most of us easily get too much in the North American diet. However, athletes with low body fat composition should take care to increase their caloric intake when they increase the frequency or duration of their sports activity.

Hydration is also incredibly important during sports activity to maintain consistent performance. Fluid requirements vary largely depending on the size of the athlete and the environmental conditions during the sports activity. We used to encourage runners to drink lots of water. Then, several runners got very sick from taking in too much water. This condition, called hyponatremia, comes from the salt composition in the blood being too diluted with water. Although rare, serious neurologic sequelae may occur in hyponatremia. As such, sports drinks were developed to replace both the salt and the water lost in the blood. Sugar was added to these drinks to increase their absorption. Some athletes get stomach cramps from the sugar and many dentists are concerned about the effects of sugar on the teeth. As such, market trends have drifted back to flavored water with sugar substitute. Regardless of which drink the athlete prefers, it is important to encourage hydration on par with losses in sweat. Water is safe to drink during sports activity, but should not be taken to excess.

Caffeinated beverages have become part of our culture in part due to desire for increased productivity at the workplace more so than on the playing field. Regardless, some athletes observe a performance effect with caffeine ingestion. The smallest dose that is effective is 250 milligrams. Side effects include restlessness, nervousness, insomnia, tremors, heightened skin sensitivity, and increased urination. Caffeine levels may be monitored in elite athletes. The permitted level of caffeine in collegiate athletics is 15 micrograms per milliliter. The permitted level in Olympic competition is 12 micrograms per milliliter.

There are two well-known regulatory bodies that have established the guidelines for what ergogenic aids are permissible in sport and at what level they are permissible. These are the NCAA and the International Olympic Committee (IOC). The NCAA has been requiring drug testing in collegiate athletes who participate in football and track since 1999. The United States Anti-Doping Agency actually runs the testing for Olympic athletes of all ages that represent the United States.

Unfortunately, most of what we have learned about ergogenic aids has come from athletes who have broken the rules. Many of these athletes have gotten very sick. In fact, the United States Anti-Doping Agency reported fifty-four potential doping violations in 2008. Prohibited substances found in the blood or urine of these athletes included anabolic agents, hormones, corticosteroids, marijuana, stimulants, medications that dilate the airways, and even a blood pressure medication.

Although most of these substances may be taken safely and legally as prescription medications in the United States, there are limits for elite athletes on the agents that may have a performance effect. For example, a patient with cancer may get shots to increase his or her red blood cell count that has decreased because of the cancer. Athletes have learned that red blood cells carry oxygen and more red blood cells may mean more oxygen delivery to the tissues. As physicians, we are aware this may have dangerous side effects. An athlete cannot have these shots unless he or she has a low red blood cell count. There is a special form that documents medical conditions in athletes. Doctors can ask for a therapeutic use exemption for the rare athlete who actually has cancer and is able to continue to compete.

The substances permitted in athletics may be very different from the substances permitted in the real world. There was a remarkable collision of permissible ergogenic aids and legal consequences in recent years in regard to Major League Baseball. Many players admitted to using anabolic steroids to get stronger. Since these players serve as role models to young boys who might be inclined to follow in their footsteps, Major League Baseball responded by creating penalties for steroid use.

Anabolic steroids are made from the male hormone, testosterone, or its relatives. Ergogenic effects include increased strength, lean muscle mass, and motivation. However, the risks of these agents far outweigh the benefits. Reversible side effects of anabolic steroids include changes in libido, decreased sperm production, scrotal pain, gynecomastia (abnormal breast growth in men), acne, hirsuitism (abnormal or excessive hair growth), edema, nervousness, aggression, liver dysfunction, nausea, and increased urination. Reversible effects may go away when the steroid is discontinued. Effects that may not go away after the steroid is discontinued include high blood pressure, changes in collagen, liver tumors, hirsuitism, voice changes, clitoral hypertrophy, premature closure of the growth plates, and psychosis. Premature closure of the growth plates may result in the athlete never achieving his expected height. Psychosis is no laughing matter as steroid use has been linked to suicide in teenagers.

Anabolic steroids come in oral and injectable forms. They have names like oxandrine and durabolin. In certain very specific cases, these agents may be used to treat medical conditions. They are not typically the first agents chosen, but they have been studied for conditions where muscle atrophy can be a life-threatening problem. For example, patients with human immunodeficiency virus (HIV) lose muscle mass as part of their disease. Steroids help increase appetite and build back muscle in those whose weight may be dangerously low. Patients with serious muscle diseases, called myopathies, may benefit from muscle-building agents. Researchers have studied the positive effect of anabolic steroids in patients with severe burn injury.

Beta-blockers are a commonly used medication to lower blood pressure. Perhaps the best-known beta blocker is metoprolol. The lower the blood pressure, the more likely an individual is to faint. Therefore, these medications would seemingly have no benefit on performance enhancement. However, these agents have a positive effect on fine motor control by decreasing anxiety. As such, they were the choice prescription for rifle sport participants. Currently, they are banned from NCAA rifle sports.

Creatine is another popular ergogenic aid that is also used in patients with certain muscle diseases. Benefits of creatine include a potential increase in biochemical factors that speed up the muscle energy pathway in the body. These effects are modest compared to anabolic steroids. As such, creatine has not received quite as much bad press. The dose to achieve this effect is 20 grams daily for five days then 5 grams daily. Most studies of creatine use have not followed the patient beyond three months. Potential adverse effects of creatine include weight gain, renal problems, and cramping.

Similar to increased protein intake, concern was raised over the ability of the normal human kidney to clear creatine. One study followed healthy athletes and found no subsequent impairment in renal function. Another report cited a case of acute renal failure after a surgical procedure in a patient taking only creatine. Debate persists on the effect of creatine on the kidney.

Cramping is a common complaint after athletic activity. Usually this is a sign of dehydration or electrolyte depletion. Electotrolytes that may play a role in cramping include calcium and potassium. When an unusually high number of athletes on creatine complained of cramping, this effect was studied in football players. No increased cramping over above that which was expected for the environmental conditions was found in players taking creatine.

Nutraceutical agents that are marketed to improve athletic performance but are not actually effective include calcium, carnitine, coenzymes Q10 and Q12, and folic acid. Promotional materials report that calcium increases muscle contractility and enhances glycogen metabolism. Although there are no data to support these claims, calcium is an important ingredient in building and maintaining healthy bones. Women tend to store the most calcium between the ages of eighteen and twenty-six so this is typically the focus group for recommendations on ingestion. The label on the carnitine bottle says that it increases fat metabolism, but this has never been proven. Coenzymes may function as antioxidants, but data are insufficient to suggest that they could improve performance. Folic acid certainly has a role in anemia and the prevention of neural tube defects in the developing fetus. However, claims that it increases aerobic capacity are unsubstantiated.

The jury is still out on whether Beta-2 agonists are effective ergogenic aids. These medications enhance smooth muscle relaxation, which leads to dilatation of the airways. For this reason, these medications are used in the treatment of asthma. Some researchers suggest that they increase lean muscle mass. However, effects on athletic performance are controversial. In the inhaled form, there has been no observed performance effect.

GENDER-BASED MEDICINE

We have known for some time that women are built differently than men. However, we are just starting to learn about how musculoskeletal injuries may be different in women. Overall, the woman's body is designed for flexibility and the man's body is designed for strength. Certainly, there are exceptions to this rule, but outward physiologic differences are apparent even in the musculoskeletal system.

In the upper limbs, women have overall less muscle bulk and strength. Women need special protection for sensitive breast tissue. Spine biomechanics in women may be affected by pendulous breasts. Women demonstrate increased flexibility of the shoulders and elbows. Further study is needed to determine if these factors affect injury rates and healing.

In the lower limbs, gender-based medicine has resulted in a successful decrease in ligamentous injury rates. Anterior cruciate ligament tears are known to be more common in women. Women have wider hips than men.

The placement of the knees relative to the hips in women puts the medial quadriceps muscle at a mechanical disadvantage. Women have weaker hamstrings than men. A focused exercise program that decreases the rate of ACL tears not only targets the quadriceps and hamstrings but teaches young women to land with their knees facing forward. This concept is illustrated in Figure 7.1.

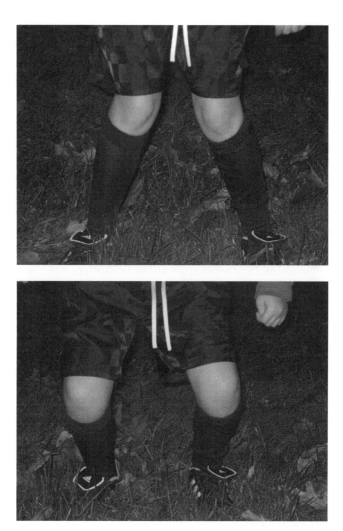

Figure 7.1. Compare the landing stance in the two images above. In the top image, the patient has landed with the knees in valgus conformation. Valgus conformation means that the knees are bending inwards. This is thought to predispose women and girls to ACL tears. In the bottom image, the patient has landed in the position recommended in ACL prevention drills. The knees are facing straight ahead. (Photos courtesy of Diane O'Brien)

The younger the athlete, the earlier good habits are formed that will hopefully last a lifetime.

Questions still remain regarding why women sustain more ligamentous injuries at the knees and ankles than men even without contact injury. Exploration of potential neuromuscular factors is underway. Further studies on the effect of female hormones on the musculoskeletal system are necessary to improve outcomes in injury and develop proper strength and conditioning programs for women.

The female hormone, estrogen, plays an important role in protection of the skeleton. Post-menopausal women are clearly at a higher risk for osteoporosis than male counterparts of the same age. With increasing age, the level of risk for osteoporosis in men approaches that of the level of risk in women. Although men do not go through menopause, testosterone levels decrease over time. The role of testosterone in bone metabolism has not been well-investigated. Perhaps, it is the increased muscle mass that prevents bone loss in men rather than a direct effect of the testosterone. Further study is necessary to clarify the role of sex hormones in bone metabolism.

NEW HORIZONS IN RESEARCH

We used to think that factors intrinsic to bone were the only factors that affected bone metabolism. Now, we know that this is no longer the case. Clinically, bone with intact overlying soft tissue heals faster from fracture than bone where the soft tissue is disrupted. Researchers have found bone loss and muscle atrophy in healthy astronauts at alarming rates even when they exercise in space. Patients with spinal cord injury experience bone loss at rates greater than normal healthy patients who are immobilized in bed. Patients with dysfunction of the sympathetic nervous system related to pain, termed complex regional pain syndrome, may exhibit relative bone loss in the area of their pain. All of these examples illustrate that there are factors at work that we may not yet completely understand in regard to bone metabolism. Healthy nerve and muscle tissue may interact with the underlying bone repair mechanisms. Research on this exciting interaction of bone with surrounding tissue would further our ability to treat such injuries.

Another exciting area of research involves the nervous system. Nerves grow back at a rate of 1 millimeter a day. This is incredibly frustrating for an athlete who is used to getting results. Mechanisms of neural repair are incompletely understood. Some cells in the nervous system simply do not regenerate. As we learn more about how nerve tissue functions, we can learn better ways to heal this tissue.

Glossary

Brachial plexus: Complicated relay station of the nerves in the shoulder that carries information to and from the arm.

Cardiologist: Doctor who specializes in the diagnosis and treatment of disorders of the heart.

Cartilage: Connective tissue covering the bones at the joint surfaces.

Computed tomography (CT): A series of x-ray-like images stacked up to get the best view of bones.

Dorsiflexion: Action of the ankle when bringing the toes toward the ceiling.

Ecchymosis: Medical term for bruise.

Edema: An abnormal accumulation of fluid in the connective tissues or body cavities.

Electrodiagnostic studies: A series of electrical pulses used to establish nerve conductivity. This is followed by a needle exam of muscles to determine the level of the nerve lesion if present.

Endocrinologist: Doctor who does residency in internal medicine and then pursues fellowship training in how hormones affect the body and how to treat metabolic abnormalities.

Ergogenic aids: Medications or food products that may enhance performance.

Ergometer: A machine used to measure the work of exercise.

Erythema: Redness of the skin caused by congestion of the blood vessels.

Estrogen: Female hormone that functions in bone remodeling.

Etiology: The cause of a disease or condition; also, the study of such causes.

Extension: Bending the limb away from the body (as in straightening the knee or the elbow).

Flexion: Bending the limb toward the body (bending the knee with the heel to buttocks or the elbow with the wrist to shoulder).

Glucocorticoids: Sugar steroids that decrease inflammation.

Hemorrhage: Bleeding into tissues after injury.

Hirsuitism: Growth of excess body hair.

Iontophoresis: Use of electric waves to encourage topical absorption of a medication (typically steroids).

Lateral: Anatomical position refers to standing forward with the arms at the sides and the palms of the hands facing forward. In this position, lateral is away from the midline of the body. For example, the lateral hand refers to the side with the thumb.

Ligament: Connective tissue that attaches one bone to another.

Magnetic Resonance Imaging (MRI): Magnetic field that creates an image which is best for viewing soft tissue inside the body.

Medial: Anatomical position refers to standing forward with the arms at the sides and the palms of the hands facing forward. In this position, medial refers to the part of the body closest to the midline. For example, the medial hand is the side with the pinky finger.

Necrosis: Death of living tissue.

Neurologist: Doctor who specializes in the diagnosis and treatment of disorders of the central and peripheral nervous system.

Orthopedic surgeon: Doctor who operates on bones, muscles, and ligaments. Many team physicians are orthopedic surgeons.

Ossification: Process by which bone stops growing and hardens to form the adult fully grown skeleton.

Osteoarthritis: Degeneration of joint surfaces that may be related to trauma, age, genetics, or unknown factors.

Osteoporosis: Loss of bone mineralization.

Palmar: Palm side of the hand.

Palpable: Able to be felt.

Phalanx: One of the bones of the fingers or the toes.

Phonophoresis: Use of ultrasound waves to encourage delivery of a topical medication, usually corticosteroids, through the skin.

Physiatrist: Doctor who specializes in returning patients to their prior function through exercise and/or pain management.

Plantar: Bottom of the foot.

Plantar flexion: Action of the ankle when pointing the toes.

Plexus: Grouping of nerves that run to different muscles and skin. For example, the brachial plexus is an interchange for the nerves of the upper limb. The lumbosacral plexus is a collection of nerves that innervates the back, pelvis, and legs.

Prognosis: What we can expect to happen with a particular disease or injury.

Prone: Lying on the stomach (face-down).

Proprioception: The ability of the mind to sense the limb's position in space.

Psychiatrist: Doctor who specializes in mental health and the diagnosis and treatment of mood disorders.

Radiographs: Also known as "plain films." Images of bone produced with radiation techniques.

Rheumatologist: Doctor who does residency in internal medicine and then pursues fellowship training in dysfunction of the body's immune system and how to treat autoimmune conditions such as rheumatoid arthritis, lupus, and psoriatic arthritis.

Sequela: Aftereffect of a disease or injury.

Soft tissue: Ligaments, tendons, muscles, and other fibrous connective tissue.

Sports: Event or activity that involves individual or team participation in a competition of athletic talents.

Sprain: Stretching or tearing of a ligament. Graded one to three depending on severity.

Strain: Stretching or tearing of a tendon. Graded one to three depending on severity.

Supine: Lying on the back (face-up).

Tendinopathy: Injury to a tendon.

Tendon: The part of the muscle that attaches to bone.

Testosterone: Male hormone that functions in building muscle.

Transcutaneous electric nerve stimulation: Topical application of electric waves used to decrease pain in soft tissue injury.

Ultrasound: Used for both diagnostic imaging and treatment of local musculo-skeletal pain.

Bibliography

BOOKS

Braddom RL. *Physical Medicine and Rehabilitation*, 2nd ed. Saunders. Philadelphia: 507–8.

Brown G. 1979. *The New York Times Encyclopedia of Sports*. Vols. 1, 2, 5, 6, 8. Football, Baseball, Golf, Tennis, and Soccer. Arno Press. New York: vii–ix. (Introduction by Frank Litsky.)

Canale ST. 1998. *Campbell's Operative Orthopedics*, 9th ed. Mosby. St Louis: 2632–33.

Danzig, A. 1956. *The History of American Football*. Prentice- Hall, Inc. Englewood Cliffs, NJ: 3–13.

Frontera, W, Silver JK, Rizzo TD. 2008. *Essentials of Physical Medicine and Rehabilitation*. Saunders/ Elsevier. Philadelphia: 315–316, 359–360, 367–8, 393–6. 271–2.

Greene WB. 2001. *Essentials of Musculoskeletal Care*, 2nd ed. American Academy of Orthopedic Surgeons. Rosemont, IL: 393–404.

Jenkins DB. 2002. *Hollinshead's Functional Anatomy of the Limbs and Back*. WB Saunders. Philadelphia: 22, 265, 279, 282, 286, 288, 306, 355–358.

Matz D. 1991. *Greek and Roman Sport*. McFarland and Company, Inc. Jefferson, NC: 5–8.

Novelline RA. 2004. *Squire's Fundamentals of Radiology*, 6th ed. Harvard University Press. Cambridge: 1–3, 29–32.

Nuland, SB. 1988. *Doctors: The Biography of Medicine*. Vintage Books. New York: 386–405.

Rockne K. 1931. *Coaching*. The Devin-Adair Company. New York: 11–12.

Sachare A. 1994. *The Official NBA Basketball Encyclopedia,* 2nd ed. Villard Books. New York: 21–23.

Thomas CL. 1997. *Taber's Cyclopedic Medical Dictionary.* F.A. Davis Company. Philadelphia: 1746.

Weinstein SL, Buckwalter JA. 2005. *Turek's Orthopedics,* 6th ed. Lippincott, Williams & Wilkins. Philadelphia: 583, 590–91.555–63.

ARTICLES

Ahrendt DM. Ergogenic aids: counseling the athlete. *Am Fam Physician.* 2001. 63:913–22.

Armas LA, Hollis BW, Heaney RP. Vitamin D2 is much less effective than vitamin D3 in humans. *J Clin Endocrinol Metab.* 2004; 89 (11):5387–91.

Balagopal P, et al. Oxandrolone enhances skeletal muscle myosin synthesis and alters global gene expression profile in Duchenne muscular dystrophy. *Am J Physiol Endocrinol Metab.* 2006 Mar; 290(3):E530–39.

Bartlett H, Eperjesi F. An ideal ocular nutritional supplement? *Ophthalmic Physiol Opt.* 2004; 24(4):339–49.

Bays HE. Safety considerations with omega-3 fatty acid therapy. *Am J Cardiol.* 2007 Mar 19; 99(6A):35C–43C. Epub 2006 Nov 28.

Biering-Sørensen F, Hansen B, Lee BS. Non-pharmacological treatment and prevention of bone loss after spinal cord injury: a systematic review. *Spinal Cord.* 2009 Jan 27.

Blumenthal M, Busse WR, Goldberg A, et al. Herb guide by pharmacologic action (approved herbs). *The Complete German Commission E monographs: Therapeutic Guide to Herbal Medicines.* The American Botanical Council, Austin TX, 1998: 462–69.

Canter PH, Wider B, Ernst E. The antioxidant vitamins A, C, E and selenium in the treatment of arthritis: a systematic review of randomized clinical trials, *Rheumatology.* 2007; 46:1223–33.

Chrubasik S, Kunzel O, Model A, et al. Treatment of low back pain with a herbal or synthetic anti-rheumatic: a randomized controlled study. Willow bark extract for low back pain. *Rheumatology.* 2001; 40:1388–93.

Clegg DO, Reda DJ, Harris CL, et al. Glucosamine, chondroitin sulfate, and the two in combination for painful knee osteoarthritis. *N Engl J Med.* 2006; 354(8):795–808.

Conn JM, Annest JL, Gilchrist J. Sports and recreation related injury episodes in the US population, 1997–99. *Inj Pre* v. 2003; 9:117–23.

Desmettre T, Lecerfe JM. [Some notions about possible harmlessness and/or toxicity of the antioxidant micronutriments.] *Bull Soc Belge Ophtalmol.* 2006; 301:25–30. French.

Dugan S. Sports-related knee injuries in female athletes. *Am J Phys Med.* 2005 Feb:122–30.

Gilchrist J, Mandelbaum BR, Melancon H, Ryan GW, et al. A randomized control trial to prevent noncontact anterior cruciate ligament injury in female collegiate soccer players. 2008 *Am J Sports Med.* 2008 Aug; 36(8):1476–83.

Greenwood M, et al. Creatine supplementation during college football training does not increase the incidence of cramping or injury. *Mol Cell Biochem.* Feb 2003.

Grennan DM, Knudson JM, Dunckley J, et al. Serum copper and zinc in rheumatoid arthritis and osteoarthritis. *N Z Med J*. 1980; 91(652):47–50.

Grunfield C, et al. Oxandrolone in the treatment of HIV-associated weight loss in men: a randomized, double-blind, placebo-controlled study. *J Acquir Immune Defic Syndr*. 2006 Mar; 41(3):304–14.

Healy WL, Sharma S, Schwartz B, et al. Athletic activity after total joint arthroplasty. *J Bone Joint Surg Amer*. 2008; 90:2245–52.

Helmick CG, Felson DT, Lawrence RC, et al. Estimates of the prevalence of arthritis and other rheumatic conditions in the United States. Part I. National Arthritis Data Workgroup. *Arthritis Rheum*. 2008 Jan; 58(1):15–25.

Hosea TM, Carey CC, Harrer MF. The gender issue: epidemiology of ankle injuries in athletes who participate in basketball. *Clin Orthop Relat Res*. 2000 Mar; 372:45–49.

Krinckas LS and Wilboum AJ. Peripheral nerve injuries in Athletes.

Kovacs FM, Abraira V, Peña A, et al. Effect of firmness of mattress on chronic nonspecific low-back pain: randomised, double-blind, controlled, multicentre trial. *Lancet*. 2003 Nov 15; 362(9396):1599–604.

Lane NE, Gore LR, Cummings SR, et al. Serum levels of vitamin D and hip osteoarthritis in elderly women: a longitudinal study, *Arthritis Rheum*. 1997; 40:S238.

McAlindon TE, Jacques P, Zhang Y, et al. Do antioxidant micronutrients protect against the development and progression of knee osteoarthritis? *Arthritis Rheum*. 1996; 39:648–56.

McAlindon TE, Felson DT, Zhang Y, et al. Relation of dietary intake and serum levels of vitamin D to progression of osteoarthritis of the knee among participants of the Framingham study. *Ann Intern Med*. 1996; 125:353–59.

McAlindon TE, Bigee BA. Nutritional factors and osteoarthritis: recent developments. *Curr Opin Rheumatol*. 2005; 17:647–52.

Nattiv A, Loucks AB, Manore MM, et al. American College of Sports Medicine Position Stand: The female athlete triad. http://www.acsm-msse.org/pt/pt-core/template-journal/msse/media/mss200785.pdf.

Newnham RE. Essentiality of boron for healthy bones & joints. *Environ Health Perspect*. 1994 Nov; 102 Suppl 7:83–85.

Newnham RE. Essentiality of boron for healthy bones and joints. Omega-3 Oil Fish or pills? *Consum Rep*. 2003; 68(7):30–32.

Payne MW, Williams DR, Trudel G. Space flight rehabilitation. *Am J Phys Med Rehabil*. 2007 Jul; 86(7):583–91.

Pietrosimone BG, Grindstaff TL, Linens SW, et al. A systematic review of prophylactic braces in the prevention of knee ligament injuries in collegiate football players. *J Athl Train*. 2008 Jul–Aug; 43(4):409–15.

Poortmans JR, Dellalieux O. Do regular high protein diets have potential health risks on kidney function in athletes? *Int J Sport Nutr Exerc Metab*. 2000 Mar; 10(1): 28–38.

Poortmans JR, Francaux M, Long-term oral creatine supplementation does not impair renal function in healthy athletes. *Med Sci Sports Ex*. 1999 Aug; 31(8):1108–10

Samuel MN, HolcombWR, Guadagnoli MA, et al. Acute effects of static and ballistic stretching on measures of strength and power. *J Strength Cond Res*. 2008 Sep; 22(5): 1422–28.

Schmid B, Ludtke R, Selbmann H, et al. Efficacy and tolerability of a standardized willow bark extract in patients with osteoarthritis: randomized placebo-controlled, double-blind clinical trial. *Phytother Res.* 2001; 15:344–50.

Schnitzer TJ. Update on guidelines for the treatment of chronic musculoskeletal pain. *Clin Rheumatol.* 2006; 25:S22–S29.

Sharma L, Song J, Felson DT, et al. The role of knee alignment in disease progression and functional decline in knee osteoarthritis. JAMA. 2001 Jul 11; 286(2):188–95.

Sheth NP, Sennet B, Berns JS. Rhabdomyolysis and ARF following arthroscopic knee surgery in a college football player taking creatine supplements *Clin Nephrol.* Feb 2006; 65(2): 134–2

Stammers T, Sibbald B, Freeling P. Efficacy of cod liver oil as an adjunct to non-steroidal anti-inflammatory drug treatment in the management of osteoarthritis in general practice. *Ann Rheum Dis.* 1992; 51:128–29.

Standaert CJ, Herring SA, Cantu RC. Expert opinion and controversies in sports and musculoskeletal medicine: concussion in the young athlete. *Arch Phys Med Rehabil.* 2007 Aug; 88(8):1077–79.

Vieth R. Vitamin D supplementation, 25-hydroxy vitamin D concentrations, and safety. *Am J Clin Nutr.* 69(5):842–56.

Volker D, Fitzgerald P, Major G, et al. Efficacy of fish oil concentrate in the treatment of rheumatoid arthritis. *J Rheumatol.* 2000; 27(10):2343–46.

Walker-Bone K. "Natural remedies" in thetreatment of osteoathritis. *Drugs Aging.* 2003; 20(7):517–26.

Wolfe SE, et al. Effects of oxandrolone on outcome measures in the severely burned: a multicenter prospective randomized double-blind trial. *J Burn Care Res.* 2006 Mar-Apr; 27(2):131–39; discussion 140–41.

Zizic TM, Marcoux C, Hungerford DS, et al. Corticosteroid therapy associated with ischemic necrosis of bone in systemic lupus erythematosus. *Am J Med.* 1985 Nov; 79(5):596–604.

OTHER CITATIONS

MMWR Weekly. September 29, 2006/ 55 (38); 1037–40.

Mundell EJ. Bengay death highlights OTC dangers. Available at www.washingtonpost.com. Accessed January 25, 2009.

Rawe J. Football's big brainteaser. *Time.* 9/17/2007. 170 (12): 58.

Reynolds G. Stretching: the truth. *The New York Times.* 11/02/2008. Available at www.nytimes.com. Accessed January 30th, 2009.

Schwartz A. Girls are often neglected victims of concussions. *The New York Times.* 10/02/2007. Available at www.nytimes.com. Accessed January 15, 2009.

Thomson's MICROMEDEX. http://www.micromedex.com. Accessed January 30, 2009.

WEB SITES

http://www.bizofbasketball.com/?option=com_content&view=article&id=395&Itemid =1 Kobritz, Jordan. Are the NCAA final four teams losing money? April 8, 2008. Accessed October, 2008.

http://www.boston.com/sports/football/patriots/articles/2008/09/11/brady_has_both_acl_
  and_mcl_tears/ Springer, Shira. Brady has both ACL and MCL tears. Accessed
  January 12, 2009.
http://college2008.upa.org/
http://www.footballbowlassociation.com/overview.html
http://www.knuterockne.com/biography.htm
http://www.littleleague.org
http://www.ncaa.org
http://www.nirsa.org
http://www.teeballusa.org
www.usada.org
http:www.usyouthsoccer.org

Index

Radius, 33, 37–38
Rheumatoid arthritis, 36
Rheumatologist, 54
Rockne, Knute, 1, 11, 21, 22, 89, 97, 113, 117
Roentgen, Wilhelm Conrad, 89
Roosevelt, Theodore, 5
Rotator cuff, 25, 28–30
Rugby, 4
Running, 16

Sacrum, 42
Salicylic acid (aspirin), 103, 110. *See also* Willow bark
Scaphoid, 37, 39
Scapula, 25–27
Sclerosis, 74
Sesamoiditis, 65
Spinal cord, 42, 45–46
Spondylolisthesis, 44–45
Spurling maneuver, 32
Steroids: anabolic steroids, 15, 119–120; corticosteroids/glucocorticoids, 12, 54, 104, 119
Stinger, 4, 32. *See also* Burner
Strawberry picker's palsy, 63
Swimming, 30

Talus, 78
Tarsal tunnel syndrome, 85

Tee ball, 12
Tennis elbow, 7, 35. *See also* Lateral epicondylitis
Testosterone, 15
Tibia, 64
Tizanidine, 51
Trapezium, 39
Trapezoid, 39
Trendelenburg sign, 59
Trigger finger, 40
Triquetrum, 39
Turf toe, 82

Ulcer/gastric ulcer, 101
Ulna, 33–34, 37
Ultimate Frisbee, 16

Valgus, 19
Vertebrae, 12, 42, 44
Vicar's knee, 72
Vitamin A, 108
Vitamin C, 108–109
Vitamin D, 80, 94, 109
Vitamin E, 108–109
Volleyball, 30

Willow bark, 110
World Series, 8
Wrestling, 10, 15, 42

About the Author

JENNIFER A. BAIMA, MD, is a clinical instructor in the Department of Physical Medicine and Rehabilitation at Harvard Medical School in Boston, Massachusetts. Dr. Baima has written extensively on the treatment of sports injuries.